Living Well with Lactose Intolerance

**JAIME ARANDA-MICHEL, M.D.
with DONALD S. VAUGHAN**

D1506243

AN AVON BOOK

The ideas, procedures, and suggestions in this book are intended to supplement, not replace, the medical advice of a trained medical professional. All matters regarding your health require medical supervision. Consult your physician before adopting the suggestions in this book, as well as about any condition that may require diagnosis or medical attention. The authors and publisher disclaim any liability arising directly or indirectly from the use of this book.

AVON BOOKS, INC.
1350 Avenue of the Americas
New York, New York 10019

Copyright © 1999 by CMD Publishing, a division of Current Medical Directions, Inc.
Illustration by Philip Ashley
Published by arrangement with CMD Publishing, a division of Current Medical Directions, Inc.
Library of Congress Catalog Card Number: 99-94790
ISBN: 0-380-80642-8
www.avonbooks.com/wholecare

First Wholecare Printing: August 1999

WHOLECARE TRADEMARK REG. U.S. PAT. OFF. AND IN OTHER COUNTRIES, MARCA REGISTRADA, HECHO EN U.S.A.

Printed in the U.S.A.

WCD   10 9 8 7 6 5 4 3 2 1

Contents

ONE

What is Lactose Intolerance?

MEET JANICE, A 33-YEAR-OLD HIGH-SCHOOL LIBRARIAN. Shortly after entering college, she began experiencing embarrassing and aggravating digestive problems after she ate—specifically stomach pain, gas, bloating, and diarrhea. At first the problem was only occasional, but as Janice aged it gradually became a daily occurrence. The symptoms usually began in the morning, and worsened as the day wore on.

"I can't really recall exactly when my problem began," Janice notes. "I've always had a sensitive stomach, but I noticed that my symptoms seemed to worsen over the past five years or so. It got to the point where I was afraid to make evening plans or go out on a date because of my condition. I never knew when the gas and diarrhea would hit, or how severe it would be. It was just horrible."

Janice visited a number of doctors, none of whom seemed able to diagnose her condition accurately. One general practitioner said she probably had an ulcer and gave her samples of a prescription ulcer medication, but it didn't help. Another doctor diagnosed her ailment as irritable bowel syndrome and recommended she go on a bland diet. But Janice found that her symptoms only got worse, so she went back to her favorite foods. A third doctor gently suggested that her problems were all in her mind and that she needed psychiatric help.

"I knew I wasn't crazy," Janice says. "I was certain there had to be a physical cause for my digestive problems, but I honestly didn't know where else to go for help. After a while I just figured it was something I was going to have to live with for the rest of my life."

Then Janice read a magazine article about a condition known as lactose intolerance, characterized by an inability to digest milk and milk products. "The more I read, the more I recognized myself," Janice recalls. "It was as if the writer were talking directly to me. I finally had an idea of what was wrong with me."

Janice quickly made an appointment with a prominent gastroenterologist in her town, who confirmed through a battery of tests that she was, indeed, lactose intolerant. Janice could comfortably digest small amounts of dairy products, but anything more was asking for trouble. With her doctor's help, Janice readjusted her lifestyle to eliminate as many dairy products as possible, and watched happily as her digestive problems all but disappeared.

"I can live a normal life again," Janice says with a laugh. "I can go out with friends and not have to worry that I'll suddenly be overcome by searing gas pains or explosive diarrhea because I ate a bowl of ice cream or drank a milkshake. I'll always have to be very careful about what I eat, but for the first time in many years, I no longer have to plan my life around the availability of rest rooms!''

Janice is far from alone. Statistics are difficult to confirm, but most researchers estimate that between 50 and 60 million Americans suffer from some degree of lactose intolerance. In fact, lactose intolerance is believed by many to be the most common genetic condition in the world—and one of the least talked about. Many people who experience mild to moderate symptoms of lactose intolerance erroneously attribute their problem to stress, an ulcer, or other digestive problems; and a sizable percentage of doctors outside of gastroenterology are unaware of how common the condition really is, how to diagnose it accurately or how to treat it. As a result, a large number of men and women spend their entire lives held hostage by a painful and frustrating condition that is actually quite easy to deal with once they know what's going on.

This book will cover all aspects of lactose intolerance, including causes, diagnostic techniques, treatment, nutrition, and lifestyle management. In this chapter, we'll talk specifically about what lactose really is, the symptoms and severity of lactose intolerance, and which populations are most at risk of developing the condition.

Q: What is lactose intolerance?
A: Lactose intolerance is a common condition characterized by the body's inability to digest milk sugar, known as lactose. This occurs because of a deficiency in the enzyme lactase, which is produced by cells that line the small intestine. Lactase breaks down lactose during the digestive process so it can be absorbed into the body. Without sufficient levels of lactase, lactose cannot be fully digested or absorbed. Undigested lactose is metab-

olized by colonic bacteria, resulting in a variety of painful symptoms, including gas, bloating, and diarrhea.

Q: Is lactose intolerance the same thing as lactose maldigestion or lactase deficiency?
A: In both cases, the answer is yes and no. Lactose maldigestion (also known as "lactose malabsorption" and "low lactose digestion capacity") is the term used by doctors if a clinical test shows that an individual does not digest all of the lactose he or she consumes, regardless of whether symptoms result. Lactase deficiency (known medically as "alactasia") is simply that—the inability to produce sufficient levels of the enzyme lactase, regardless of the cause or the appearance of symptoms. Lactose intolerance (commonly known outside of the United States as "hypolactasia" or "lactase restriction") is a condition characterized by the appearance of noticeable digestive symptoms after the ingestion of lactose-containing dairy products.

There are some slight clinical differences between the above terms, but to the layperson they're all essentially the same. For the purpose of this book, we'll use the phrase "lactose intolerance" as an umbrella term when discussing symptoms resulting from the inability to digest dairy products because of a lactase deficiency.

Q: Is lactose intolerance a disease? Can it be cured?
A: Lactose intolerance is not a disease. It's a condition that occurs naturally, and for most people is simply a part of aging. It's not something that you can catch from others, like the flu, though there is a genetic component—people with the most common form of lactose intolerance, known as primary acquired lactose intolerance, are likely to have inherited a gene from their par-

ents that causes their bodies to stop producing lactase.

Because lactose intolerance is not a disease, it cannot be prevented; nor can it be cured in the traditional sense of the word. However, it can be easily managed through some simple changes in diet and lifestyle, which we'll discuss later in this book.

Q: Is being born with lactose intolerance the only way to get the condition, or can it be triggered by other things?

A: Primary acquired lactose intolerance is by far the most common form of the condition, but lactase production can also be affected by other things, such as intestinal disease or surgery. This is known as secondary lactose intolerance (SLI). We'll discuss the varied causes of lactose intolerance in greater detail in Chapter Two.

Q: Is lactose intolerance the same thing as a milk allergy?

A: No. Many people mistakenly assume that being lactose intolerant is the same thing as being allergic to milk, but they are actually two completely different medical conditions. Lactose intolerance is an enzyme deficiency— the body doesn't produce enough of the enzyme lactase to break down lactose properly in the intestines. A true milk allergy is an immune response in which the body produces antibodies to cow's milk protein (CMP). The symptoms and treatments of each disorder are decidedly different. (See Chapter Three for a more detailed discussion of milk allergy.)

Q: Could you give us a little more information on lactose? For example, how is it formed and how common is it in our diets?

A: Lactose is a compound sugar made by combining two simple sugars known as glucose and galactose. It is a member of the carbohydrate family, as are other naturally occurring sugars such as fructose, sucrose, and maltose. During the digestion process, lactose is broken down into its component parts by the enzyme lactase and used as energy for the body, or stored in the form of glycogen for later use. When glycogen is very plentiful, it is converted by the body into fat for long-term storage.

All milk, regardless of what animal it comes from, contains lactose. And because cow's milk is an ingredient in many types of foods, lactose is extremely common in the traditional American diet. You can find it almost everywhere—in milk, ice cream, cheese, and any product made with whole milk or milk products. The widespread use in the United States of milk and milk products in foods can make life miserable for people who are severely lactose intolerant; in many cases, even a tiny amount of lactose can produce painful symptoms. As a result, people with lactose intolerance must spend a lot of time making sure the foods they eat are low-lactose or lactose-free, or take special enzyme pills to help them digest lactose more easily.

Q: Glucose and galactose, the simple sugars that combine to make lactose, sound like important nutrients. Is it unhealthy to deprive the body of them by avoiding milk products?

A: You have nothing to worry about. Glucose is a vital source of energy for the human body, but you're not doing yourself any harm by cutting back on dairy products because *all* of the carbohydrates in your diet are converted into glucose during the digestive process. As for galactose, it's relatively unimportant on its own, serving only to bind with glucose to form lactose. Bottom line: As long as you maintain a healthy diet that includes plenty of fresh fruits and vegetables, you should have few nutrition problems. Most of the other essential nutrients found in milk products, such as calcium, vitamin D, and protein, can also be obtained through nondairy sources as well as commercial supplements. We'll discuss this issue in greater detail in Chapter Six: Maintaining Proper Nutrition with Lactose Intolerance.

Q: How much glucose do we have in our bodies at a given time? Since it's an essential fuel, I would imagine that our bodies have large stores of the stuff.

A: You're in for a big surprise—most of us have just one-fifth of an ounce of glucose in our bloodstreams at any one time. Blood glucose feeds energy-starved cells whenever they need it, but the human body is one of the most efficient machines in existence, so a tiny amount goes a very long way.

The body, as you might imagine, is very energy intensive and needs a lot of fuel to maintain itself. It must repair damaged cells, as well as run the digestive, circulatory, and other essential systems. Blood glucose levels are depleted approximately every 15 minutes, so the body replenishes its fuel supply by turning to reserve stores in the form of glycogen, which is broken down into glucose in a process known as glycolysis.

Q: What are the most common symptoms of lactose intolerance?

A: There are many, but the most common are bloating, cramps, rumbling in the gut (known medically as borborygmi), flatulence, nausea, and diarrhea following the consumption of milk, milk products, or foods made with milk products. Of course, these symptoms vary from individual to individual and not everyone experiences all of them. Children, for example, may vomit as a symptom of lactose intolerance, but this is relatively rare in adults.

There are also a variety of secondary problems associated with lactose intolerance and the avoidance of dairy products. The most common is a calcium deficiency, which can lead to weak, brittle bones. And while relatively rare, certain nutritional disorders may result from an avoidance of dairy products, such as rickets, fatigue, and a weakened immune system.

The intensity of primary symptoms and the length of time before they are felt depends on a number of factors, including the severity of the condition (i.e. the amount of lactase produced in the intestines), the amount of lactose that has been consumed, and whether or not it was consumed with other foods. A small glass of milk may result in only mild symptoms (or no symptoms at all) in people with a moderate form of the condition, especially if consumed with a meal, whereas the same amount could cause immediate and explosive symptoms in very severe cases. Everyone is different, but as a rule of thumb, bloating is typically experienced approximately 15 to 30 minutes after consuming a specific amount of lactose, with abdominal pain and flatulence striking within one to two hours. However, it's not uncommon for individuals to feel the effects of lactose ingestion several hours after the fact. Symptoms usually last only a few hours, though they may persist for a day or more in extremely sensitive individuals. It all depends on how long it takes a particular food to work its way through the digestive tract.

It's interesting to note that while the phrase "lactose intolerance" didn't make it into American medical literature until the 1960s, the problem was first recognized thousands of years ago. Hippocrates, the Greek physician who has come to be known as the father of medicine, noted that "milk is bad for patients with fever, those whose bellies are distended and full of rumbling." And six hundred years later, Galen, a Roman of Greek heritage whose concepts influenced medical thinking for centuries, accurately noted the dangers of milk consumption among those who could not digest it. "Milk should not be given to all, but only those who digest it well," Galen stated. "If sometimes it should ever be taken alone without bread, it both goes through more quickly and is flatulent. But somebody was sick all the time, no matter in what way he prepared it. And somebody else, similarly trying to use the milk, had no trouble, for he digested it well, and had no hyperacidity, or eructation or gas."

Over the years, other authorities noted the physical problems that often accompanied milk consumption, though milk continued to be a widely used source of nutrition in many cultures. Around 1860, German researchers found that milk sugar (later known as lactose) gave dogs diarrhea, and by the 1890s, scientists were well aware of the existence of the enzyme lactase in the intestines and the fact that only young animals demonstrated lactase activity.

By the turn of the century the detrimental effects of lactose in people had become more widely recognized. In 1900, Abraham Jacobi, professor of the Diseases of Children at Columbia University, gave one of the first speeches on the dangers of milk sugar to the Children's Section of the Thirteenth International Medical Congress. In his talk, Jacobi encouraged pediatricians to use cane sugar rather than milk sugar to sweeten cow's milk because milk sugar was widely known to cause diarrhea. In fact, so strong were milk sugar's effects on the digestive system that it was often used to unblock constipated infants. But despite the efforts of Jacobi and others, the adverse effects of lactose consumption were largely ignored by the medical profession for several more decades.

Q: My cousin is HIV-positive and has been experiencing frequent diarrhea and other digestive problems. Is it possible that his symptoms could be caused by lactose intolerance?

A: It's possible, but your cousin should consult his doctor for a lactose-intolerance test to be sure. If he has only recently been experiencing digestive symptoms, it's more likely that he's got an infection of the gastrointestinal tract or is experiencing side effects from his medications, both of which are extremely common among people with HIV.

To tentatively confirm a diagnosis of lactose intolerance, your cousin should avoid all lactose-containing products for three or four days and monitor his symptoms. If they seem to get better during this period, lactose intolerance may be the cause of his problems. But again, your cousin should consult his physician for a more accurate diagnosis. If laboratory tests absolutely confirm lactose intolerance, his doctor can help him formulate a healthy dietary management plan.

Q: What happens in the digestive system to cause the symptoms most commonly seen among people who

are lactose intolerant? Why is a lactase deficiency such a problem?

A: As noted earlier, the body needs lactase to break down lactose into its component parts for easy absorption. If there are insufficient levels of lactase to do the job, then the undigested lactose stays in the intestines, where it causes all sorts of problems.

For example, undigested lactose is thick so it dilutes itself by pulling water from surrounding tissue into the small intestine, resulting in distention and the painful bloating so common in lactose-intolerance sufferers. The watery mix pushes its way deeper into the digestive tract until it reaches the colon, which is unable to absorb large amounts of water. It's in the colon, too, that the undigested lactose comes in contact with normally beneficial intestinal bacteria, which view the material as a tasty smorgasbord. The hungry organisms break down the mix through fermentation, and in the process produce large amounts of carbon dioxide, which can cause additional discomfort and embarrassing rumbling noises in your gut. But that's not all. The excess liquid and gas put increasing pressure on the colon, sometimes resulting in explosive watery diarrhea and flatulence. In very severe cases, victims may not even be able to control bowel function and may soil themselves.

It may sound like a joke to some, but lactose intolerance is no laughing matter. People with severe forms of the condition report that the resulting gas and other symptoms can be so painful as to be incapacitating, and that the condition dramatically affects the quality of their lives.

Q: How common is lactose intolerance?

A: That really depends on who you talk to. Some researchers believe it's extremely common, afflicting the vast majority of adults worldwide. Others believe the numbers aren't quite so high, though they do admit that lactose maldigestion is probably more common than most doctors realize. It's often stated that more than 50 million North Americans are lactose intolerant to some degree, as are an equal or greater number of Europeans. That's probably pretty close to the truth. However, many people with mild to moderate lactose intolerance may go their entire lives without ever being properly diagnosed because their symptoms are not severe enough for them to seek medical help.

Q: Why is lactose intolerance so common? It's as if nature were intentionally trying to keep us away from dairy products.

A: In a way, you're right. It's been speculated that primary acquired lactose intolerance, the most common form of the condition, is nature's way of weaning children off milk and onto solid foods. It may sound odd, but it's a theory supported by medical evidence. For example, our ability to digest milk starts to wane very shortly after we're born. Lactase levels are high after birth because mother's milk is an infant's primary food source, but begin to decline as solid foods are introduced. In most cases, lactase production has slowed considerably by the time a child is off milk completely, and will continue to dwindle the rest of the individual's life. The continued consumption of milk and milk products does nothing to influence lactase production, and in sensitive individuals only results in painful symptoms.

Q: Are some people more prone to lactose intolerance? Does it afflict certain groups more than others?

A: Most definitely. Lactose intolerance is a global condition, though it afflicts certain populations much more commonly than others. Statistics vary, but many researchers believe that as many as 95 percent of African blacks, Asians, and Dravidian Indians are lactose intolerant to some degree. Also very commonly afflicted are American Indians, South and Central American Indians, Mexican Americans and North American blacks. In addition, between 60 and 90 percent of people of Mediterranean heritage are lactose intolerant, as are up to 75 percent of Jews of Eastern European heritage.

Those less affected, researchers say, are Middle Europeans (10 to 20 percent), Northern Europeans (1 to 5 percent), North American whites (15 to 20 percent) and Northwestern Indians of India and Pakistan (3 to 15 percent). For these groups, lactose intolerance is an unusual medical condition, whereas it's the norm for the rest of the world's population.

Why are some people less likely to develop lactose intolerance than others? That's a question scientists are still trying to figure out. The ability to digest lactose is a relatively new development; researchers believe that until very recently—maybe 10,000 years ago—almost everyone in the world was lactose intolerant.

One popular theory is that those groups which currently exhibit a strong tolerance to dairy products are the lucky recipients of thousands of years of natural selection. In areas where dairy products were a plentiful and much-used source of nutrition, such as northern Europe and parts of what is now India and Pakistan, those who were able to tolerate lactose survived better than those who were not, so their lactose-tolerant genes were passed down from one generation to the next. Those who can safely consume milk and other dairy products today are merely part of a long line of lactose-tolerant individuals.

The gradual mixing of populations and races has obviously benefited certain groups. For example, almost all West African blacks are lactose intolerant, yet only around 75 percent of American blacks are unable to consume dairy products. The remaining 25 percent or so have received lactose-tolerant genes as a result of interracial mixing over the years. Similar cases can be found in other areas of the world as well.

Q: If the vast majority of lactose intolerance is genetic, why am I lactose intolerant yet my parents are not? That doesn't make sense. Shouldn't they also be unable to digest lactose?

A: In theory, yes. But genetics is a numbers game that occasionally throws us a curve. First, you have to understand that lactase production is controlled by a gene on the second of the 46 pairs of chromosomes found in all human beings. There are two forms of the gene, one that makes us lactose tolerant (which we'll call LT), and one that makes us lactose intolerant (which we'll call LI).

One set of each pair of genes comes from our mothers, and one set comes from our fathers. As a result, the pair we're born with can be one of only four potential combinations: LT (from your mother) and LT (from your father); LI (mother) and LI (father); LT (mother) and LI (father); and LI (mother) and LT (father). The lactose tolerant (LT) gene is dominant and the lactose intolerant

(LI) gene is recessive. So people who have an LT/LI combination will always be lactose tolerant and thus able to digest dairy products without a problem.

In your particular case, the most probable explanation is that both of your parents had an LI/LT combination, which meant that (since LT is always dominant) they were able to digest lactose properly and you received an LI gene from both your mother and your father. The result: LI/LI or lactose intolerance.

Q: How serious is lactose intolerance in comparison to other digestive diseases? Can it lead to more serious illnesses?
A: In the big picture, lactose intolerance is little more than an inconvenience. True, the symptoms of severe lactose intolerance can have a detrimental impact on an individual's lifestyle, but once the condition is accurately diagnosed and the person learns how to manage his diet properly, the condition should become a minor concern at best.

Lactose intolerance by itself does not appear to lead to more serious forms of intestinal illness, though its symptoms, if not controlled, can result in a number of potentially dangerous health problems. Chronic diarrhea, for example, can quickly lead to severe dehydration and related complications, especially in young children, the elderly, and individuals whose immune systems have been compromised by illness. In addition, gas and bloating can be so excruciating that the victim can barely move. And the complete exclusion of all milk products in a desperate attempt to avoid symptoms can cause a calcium deficiency and other nutritional disorders if not corrected with healthful, nondairy alternatives and dietary supplements.

Q: I've lived with moderate lactose intolerance for several years and try to watch my diet, though occasionally a lactose-containing food slips by. Is there anything I can do to counter the effects once symptoms start to manifest themselves?

A: Not really. The standard treatments for the most common symptoms of lactose intolerance don't work very well because of the unique nature of the condition. Antacids, for example, are fairly useless because they are made to neutralize stomach acid, not intestinal gas. Over-the-counter diarrhea medications may sound like a good idea, but there's a good chance they'll only prolong your agony. Rather than halting the process, which most diarrhea medications are designed to do, it's better to get the lactose, bacteria, and water out of your system as quickly as you can. In most cases, medication should be taken only for residual diarrhea after you're sure the undigested lactose is long gone.

Antigas medications, such as those containing the drug simethicone, may be effective in relieving the flatulence that commonly afflicts the lactose intolerant, but there are no guarantees. Simethicone and similar compounds make gas easier to expel, but they don't really tackle the cause of the problem.

There is some evidence that taking lactase supplements, such as Lactaid, at the very first sign of symptoms may help reduce their severity. But again, there are no promises. These enzyme-containing digestion aids work best when taken before and during lactose-rich meals, but if you forget, it can't hurt to pop a couple immediately after. (See Chapter Four: How is Lactose Intolerance Treated? for more information on the use and effectiveness of lactase supplements.)

Perhaps someday someone will create a pill that will

quickly and effectively neutralize all of the symptoms of lactose intolerance. But until then, the best you can do is let the symptoms run their course, try a little harder to keep lactose-containing foods out of your diet, and take lactase supplements when you know you'll be consuming lactose.

Q: What specific digestive problems could indicate lactose intolerance? I suffer from occasional gas after meals and at other times, but I never really thought that I could be lactose intolerant. Now I'm not so sure.

A: Gas is one of the most common indicators of lactose intolerance. It's also one of the most easily dismissed. Most gastroenterologists who deal frequently with lactose intolerance will tell you that, as a rule of thumb, gas or intestinal rumblings that routinely follow a meal should be considered lactose-based until a lactose intolerance test proves otherwise. If it happens only occasionally and is not accompanied by any of the other symptoms that typically indicate lactose intolerance, it's probably caused by something else.

Gas that hits every day and gets worse as the day progresses is another strong indicator of lactose intolerance. So is chronic, unexplained diarrhea—especially if it usually occurs within an hour after eating. And of course, if you're a non-Caucasian experiencing these symptoms, the possibility of lactose intolerance is even stronger.

Q: I have many of the symptoms of lactose intolerance. Should I automatically assume that I have the condition?

A: No. Having some of the symptoms of lactose intolerance doesn't necessarily mean you're lactose intolerant. Many diseases—some of them quite serious—and other medical conditions have similar symptoms, so it's unwise to base your self-diagnosis only on that. Instead, consult a gastroenterologist for a proper medical workup. He'll give you the appropriate tests and confirm once and for all whether you're truly lactose intolerant. (See Chapter Five for a discussion of diseases and conditions that can mimic lactose intolerance).

Q: A friend of mine who was recently diagnosed with lactose intolerance told me that you don't have to exhibit obvious symptoms to be lactose intolerant. Is that true? If so, how would you know you have the condition?

A: Lactose intolerance is a funny condition in that it's not black-and-white; there are a lot of gray areas when it comes to symptoms, diagnosis, and management. For example, some people who test positive for lactose intolerance can drink a fair amount of milk and never experience a single symptom, while others who test negative may still be very sensitive to certain dairy products. In addition, some people who are lactose intolerant experience symptoms every day, while others may have problems only occasionally.

The reasons for this bizarre disparity are many, doctors say. It's important to realize that no one is completely lactase deficient. With very rare exceptions, we all produce a small amount of this important enzyme, which means that we can digest at least a little lactose every day. It's only when we exceed a specific amount that we experience the condition's telltale symptoms.

In addition, some foods with lactose are much easier to digest than others. A good example is yogurt, which is certainly a dairy product but which most people with lactose intolerance find easy to digest because of its bacterial cultures. It's also possible that some people are able to tolerate a certain amount of lactose-containing foods because they eat them regularly. Such people may experience minimal symptoms, but they are so mild as to be almost unnoticeable.

Q: Is there anything a person with lactose intolerance can do to stimulate the production of lactase? That seems like the easiest way to remedy the condition.
A: If only it were that simple! Sadly, once our bodies start to limit lactase production, there's very little we can do about it. A reduction in lactase production is a natural physical phenomenon that cannot be influenced by medication, herbs, or anything else. We can't even affect the rate of decrease—in most cases it's established genetically. Symptoms can be managed through proper diet, but once you're lactose intolerant, it's likely you'll always be lactose intolerant.

Q: Does everyone with primary acquired lactose intolerance stop producing lactase at the same time, or is everyone different?
A: For the most part, everyone's different. Some individuals may stop producing sufficient amounts of lactase before their first birthday, while others may maintain adequate levels until they stop ''weaning'' (move from milk to solid foods exclusively)—traditionally around age 4 or 5, though in the United States it usually occurs much earlier. The majority of people experience a decline in lactase production so gradual that they don't begin to experience symptoms until adulthood, and a few hardy souls are able to consume all the milk products they want well into their senior years. Finally, there are

those lucky few who never stop producing lactase and can ingest large amounts of milk products right up until the end.

Because of the individuality of this condition, there is no typical age for the onset of lactose intolerance; you might start noticing symptoms at age 5 or age 75. For most people, however, the symptoms of lactose intolerance become a noticeable concern in middle age. Typically, that's when lactase production has slowed to the point where lactose can no longer be tolerated in normal amounts.

Q: After years of worsening symptoms, I've been diagnosed with lactose intolerance. I'm disheartened by this news because I really like certain dairy items, such as cottage cheese and ice cream. Must I avoid all dairy products? Will everything containing milk result in symptoms?

A: That's a difficult question to answer because, as noted earlier, lactose intolerance is not an all-or-nothing disease. There are a number of factors to consider in determining what you can and cannot eat, the most important being the severity of your condition. If your condition is relatively minor, you should be able to consume at least small amounts of just about anything you want. But if it's severe, you may find your diet strictly limited in regard to dairy products, though lactase supplements and dairy-free substitutes can be quite beneficial. People with severe lactose intolerance should also investigate international cuisines that don't rely as much on milk products as American foods do. Most Asian dishes, for example, incorporate very few dairy products, often substituting soy milk or soy products in place of cow's milk.

Most people with lactose intolerance, however, find

that they can digest some dairy products more easily than others, and that's probably true of you, too. Milk is packed with lactose (an 8-ounce glass contains approximately 12 grams of lactose) and most people with lactose intolerance can drink only small amounts, if any, without exhibiting symptoms. But butter and some aged cheeses are fairly low in lactose and easily tolerated by people with mild to moderate forms of the condition. And almost all people with lactose intolerance can consume yogurt with very few problems.

Determining how much of your favorite dairy products you can safely eat will require some trial and error. Start with very small amounts and gradually increase them until you start to feel the onset of symptoms.

"I really love ice cream and I thought my life was over when my doctor confirmed that I had lactose intolerance," notes Angela, a 44-year-old executive secretary. "The idea of never being able to eat my favorite kinds of ice cream again was very depressing. After a lot of searching I finally found a brand that was lactose-reduced, but I didn't find it as satisfying. It just didn't taste right to me.

"During my annual checkup, my doctor informed me that my lactose intolerance was only in the low-to-moderate range, and that I should still be able to enjoy my favorite brands of ice cream as long as I was careful. I started with a single spoonful and rejoiced when nothing happened. A couple of days later I upped the ante to half a serving—and again I felt fine. But when I added another couple of scoops, my gut told me I had crossed the line. I now enjoy a small bowl of ice cream every evening after dinner. It's not as much as I would like, but at least it's something. Just because you have lactose intolerance doesn't necessarily mean you have to give up on every dairy product. You simply need to use some common sense and listen to your body."

Q: Does being lactase-deficient always mean a person will be lactose intolerant?
A: Since lactose intolerance is caused by a reduction in lactase production, the logical answer should be yes. But the clinical answer, as noted earlier, is "not always." It's possible to be lactase-deficient but not lactose intolerant. Though related, they're really two separate issues. A diagnosis of lactose intolerance is made when the incomplete absorption of lactose, as measured by a rise in breath hydrogen levels, is accompanied by gastrointestinal symptoms, including gas, bloating, and diarrhea. But not everyone who is lactase-deficient experiences the telltale symptoms of lactose intolerance.

Michael Levitt, MD, director of research at the Minneapolis Veterans Affairs Medical Center, confirmed in a recent randomized, double-blind crossover study that not all lactase-deficient individuals are lactose intolerant.

Levitt recruited 30 adults who believed they were severely lactose intolerant. Tests showed that nine members of the group produced some level of lactase, while 21 did not. All of the subjects were asked to drink eight ounces of milk with breakfast for two weeks. One week the milk was treated so lactose could be easily digested, the next week it was not.

"A good share of the subjects thought they would have to withdraw from the study because they wouldn't be able to tolerate the milk we were asking them to drink," Levitt noted. "However, no one in the test noticed more stomach problems from the regular milk than the lactose-reduced (brand)."

Levitt and colleagues concluded in the resulting *New*

England Journal of Medicine report that when lactose intake is limited to eight ounces or less a day, symptoms are likely to be insignificant. They stressed, however, that their findings were based on adults and should not be extrapolated to children.

A second double-blind study published in the *American Journal of Clinical Nutrition* found similar results. Finnish researchers Tuula H. Vesa, Riita A. Korpela, and Timo Sahi recruited 39 people who had trouble digesting lactose and 15 who did not. All were placed on a lactose-free diet, and every third day they were given a glass of milk containing 0, 0.5, 1.5 or 7.5 grams of lactose. The occurrence and severity of symptoms, if any, were recorded over the 12 hours following consumption.

The lactose maldigesters reported more bloating as lactose levels increased, but there was no significant difference in the mean severity of symptoms and nearly one-third of the maldigesters reported no symptoms at all. Interestingly, the same number of maldigesters reported symptoms after drinking lactose-free milk as with that containing the highest lactose content. Concluded the researchers: "Our results seem to indicate that an entirely lactose-free diet is only rarely necessary."

Q: I'm trying to figure out just how dramatically my lactose intolerance will affect my normal diet. Could you provide a few examples of dairy products that are high in lactose and others that are relatively low?

A: Certainly. Foods known to have a very high lactose content include all varieties of cow's milk, including whole, low-fat, extra-light, powdered, evaporated, non-fat, and chocolate; whipping cream and sour cream; ice cream; all cheeses except those that have aged for 90 days or more (aging greatly reduces lactose content); hot chocolate and other flavored powdered beverages that contain milk powder; powdered and liquid coffee creamers (except those specifically labeled "nondairy"); instant breakfast drinks; desserts made with milk, pudding, or custard; and cream sauces on foods.

Dairy products relatively low in lactose include lactose-reduced milk, sweet acidophilus milk, yogurt, and frozen yogurt desserts. Sherbet, while not technically a dairy dessert, is often lumped with ice cream. It, too, is very low in lactose.

Dietary management tips, including a more thorough discussion of "hidden" lactose, can be found in Chapter Seven.

Q: I've been reading a lot lately about gene therapy, in which specific genes are manipulated to prevent or correct a particular medical condition. Could gene therapy be used to help people with lactose intolerance?

A: Not at the moment, though gene therapy certainly holds some promise. According to a report in the journal *Nature Medicine*, researchers in the United States and New Zealand recently were able to induce greater lactose tolerance in rats by injecting a gene that directs the production of lactase directly into the animals' digestive tracts.

That's good news for lactose-intolerant rats, but we humans shouldn't get our hopes up too high. Years of work will be required before doctors can even begin to talk about gene therapy as a possible cure for lactose intolerance in people. Besides, there are many medical problems more serious than lactose intolerance that would no doubt benefit more from this astounding scientific advance.

Q: You mentioned earlier that lactose can be found in the milk of all mammals. How does the lactose content of cow's milk compare with that of other animals? Would goat's milk be a safer substitute?
A: On a chart showing the lactose levels of various animal milks, cow's milk would fall somewhere in the middle with an average lactose content of 3.7 to 5.1 percent, say zoologists. Some mammals have decidedly less lactose in their milk, and others have decidedly more. Porpoise milk, for example, contains only 1.3 percent lactose, and mink milk only 2.0 percent. Elephant milk, on the other hand, may contain between 4.7 and 8.8 percent lactose. However, size isn't necessarily a good corollary of lactose percentages. Whale milk—which is produced by some of the largest mammals on Earth—contains an average of only 1.8 percent lactose.

Goat's milk is consumed by numerous cultures around the world, but it's not a particularly good substitute for people with lactose intolerance because it can contain up to 4.7 percent lactose—as much as cow's milk.

As for human milk, it contains even more lactose than cow's milk with an average of 6.2 to 7.5 percent.

Q: Is all mammal's milk the same? In other words, is human breast milk essentially the same as cow's milk?
A: Not really. The nutritional content of a particular milk depends on that animal's specific needs. These are influenced by a number of factors, including the animal's size and the climate and terrain of its natural habitat. Human breast milk contains approximately 6.9 percent

lactose, 4.6 percent fat, 1.23 percent protein and 73 calories per 100 grams. Reindeer milk, in comparison, contains 2.4 percent lactose, 22.50 percent fat, 10.30 percent protein and a whopping 250 calories per 100 grams. That's because reindeer are indigenous to a very cold and inhospitable climate and require a lot more calories to survive. The fat content in reindeer milk is considerably higher than in human breast milk because fat contains more calories.

While we Americans are accustomed to drinking cow's milk only, many other cultures prefer the milk of other animals, such as goats, reindeer, and even camels. Historians note that horse milk, which contains twice the vitamin C of human breast milk and four times that of cow's milk, was no doubt the nutritional savior of the nomadic Mongols of Asia, whose diet contained very, very few fruits or vegetables. Malnutrition and related diseases would almost certainly have wiped them out had the Mongols been a cattle-based people. Instead, their culture revolved around the horse, which provided essential nutrients as well as transportation.

(See Chapter Eight: Lactose Intolerance and Special Populations for more information on breast milk and its effects on lactose-intolerant babies.)

TWO

What are the Causes of
Lactose Intolerance?

JOHN AND KEN HAVE BEEN THE BEST OF FRIENDS SINCE the second grade, when Ken's family moved to John's hometown. Kindred spirits from the very beginning, they grew up to share an avid interest in baseball and fast cars, played sports together in high school, and even went to the same college, where they met and married twin sisters. John and Ken were inseparable almost their entire lives, and their friendship is as strong today as it was when they first met.

In addition to their continued interest in baseball and sports cars, John and Ken share a very common medical problem—lactose intolerance. But they developed the condition in decidedly different ways.

John first noticed the onset of digestive symptoms as a freshman in college. At first the gas and bloating, which almost always occurred shortly after he ate, was relatively mild, and John paid it little attention. But over time the symptoms worsened. By his junior year, John could no longer consume many of his favorite foods, including chocolate ice cream and strawberry milk shakes, without experiencing extreme gastrointestinal distress.

Worried that he might be seriously ill, John visited a doctor on campus, who referred him to a gastroenterologist. After John described his symptoms, the doctor performed several tests and, much to John's relief, confirmed a diagnosis of primary acquired lactose intolerance. John learned how to manage his condition with a low-lactose diet, and is still able to enjoy small portions of his favorite dairy foods.

Ken, on the other hand, was one of those rare individuals who, thanks to a genetic fluke, was able to consume as much lactose as he liked without experiencing a single symptom. While John was forced to monitor his diet carefully, Ken could enjoy two glasses of milk and a heaping bowl of ice cream and never feel a thing.

Shortly after graduating from college, Ken developed a severe intestinal infection of the lower intestine following a Mexican vacation with his fiancée. He complained of persistent nausea, severe diarrhea, and a burning fever coupled with chills. When the problem didn't go away after two days, Ken's fiancée rushed him to the hospital, where his condition was diagnosed and treatment started. He was released three days later.

A health nut, Ken recovered fairly quickly from the incident and tried to put it behind him. But almost immediately he noticed a lingering aftereffect—painful bloating, rumbling gas, and sudden diarrhea whenever he ate dairy products. Ken consulted his doctor, who informed him that he had developed secondary lactose intolerance; the severe intestinal infection had apparently affected his body's ability to produce sufficient levels of lactase. No longer would he be able to enjoy heaping bowls of ice cream or other dairy products. At least, not in the quantities he had before. Like his best friend John, Ken now had to follow a low-lactose diet or suffer the consequences.

The vast majority of lactose-intolerance cases are the result of a conspiracy between age and genetics. But the condition can also be triggered by a number of other factors, including injury and disease. In this chapter, we'll discuss the digestive process, all of the major causes of lactose intolerance, temporary forms of the condition, and, where applicable, its possible prevention.

Q: Since lactose intolerance is considered a digestive disorder, could you offer a simple overview of the human digestive system? In order to understand how digestive problems occur, I think it's necessary to understand the normal process.
A: Most people take digestion for granted, and don't give it much thought. They eat, the food gets digested, and then they eliminate the waste. But in truth, digestion is a complex, multistage process that proves what an amazing and efficient machine the human body really is.

The path from the mouth to the anus is known medically as the alimentary canal. Think of it as a road with many stops along the way—the esophagus, the stomach, the small intestine, the large intestine (also known as the colon), the rectum, and the anus. The very first stop, obviously, is the mouth. It's there that food is chewed and mixed with saliva, which begins the digestive process by breaking down starches. From the mouth, food is passed down the throat, through the esophagus, and into the stomach. Many people believe their stomach is located around their belly button, but it actually can be found just a little below the heart, protected by the first five ribs on your rib cage.

The stomach is an amazing organ. Empty, it's surprisingly small. But it's also very flexible and, if pushed to the limit, can hold up to two quarts of food and water. However, forcing that much food into the stomach, as we often do on many holidays, can be very uncomfortable. In the stomach, food is mixed with digestive juices and "mulched" into tiny pieces by muscle contractions. The end result is a watery soup known medically as chyme. Anyone who has ever vomited knows what it looks like.

The primary component of stomach juice is hydrochloric acid, one of the most corrosive substances known. The stomach produces a weak 0.5 percent solution of hydrochloric acid, but it's still pretty potent. If you were to get some on your skin, it would cause a painful burn. The stomach protects itself by secreting a substance called mucin, which adheres to the stomach lining as a thick layer of mucous. If this layer cracks or is otherwise reduced, painful gastric ulcers may result. A reduction in mucin production occurs with age, which is why gastric ulcers tend to afflict the elderly more than other age groups. Once food has been turned into chyme, it is pushed from the stomach into the small intestine through the pyloric sphincter. Liquids usually pass through very quickly, while solid matter may take several hours.

It's in the small intestine that digestion really begins. The key is millions of tiny projections known as villi, which absorb available nutrients as the chyme slowly makes it way through. The small intestine is about 23 feet in length and is divided into three sections: the duodenum, the jejunum, and the ileum. The duodenum and the jejunum connect at a sharp angle known as the ligament of Trietz, which is where lactose production is highest in the small intestine.

Interestingly, the duodenum is the smallest section of the small intestine, but easily the most important to the digestive process. Almost all digestion takes place there, except for that of sugars, which occurs in the jejunum. If problems occur in the duodenum via injury or disease, digestion can be seriously impaired.

Though less than a foot in length, the duodenum works extremely hard. Acidic chyme empties into it all day long, but the duodenum doesn't have the same protective coating as the stomach, so it must look elsewhere for protection. Its saviors are the liver, gallbladder, and pancreas, which provide the duodenum with alkaline bile salts and pancreatic juice, all of which help neutralize stomach acid so the duodenum doesn't get burned. The pancreatic juices also help digest proteins, starches, and fats so the chyme can move into the jejunum. Reduced acid levels in the duodenum signal the pyloric sphincter to open up and pour more acidic chyme into the duodenum. This process is repeated for several hours following every meal.

Additional digestive enzymes are released in the jejunum. To us, the most important are the disaccharidases, which split compound sugars (disaccharides) into simple sugars. As you may have guessed, lactase is a disaccharide, so it's here that lactose is finally broken down into glucose and galactose and absorbed into the body via the villi in the jejunum. (At least in people with sufficient levels of lactase.)

The third leg of our trip through the small intestine is the ileum, which is responsible for absorbing a number of important nutrients, including bile salts and certain B

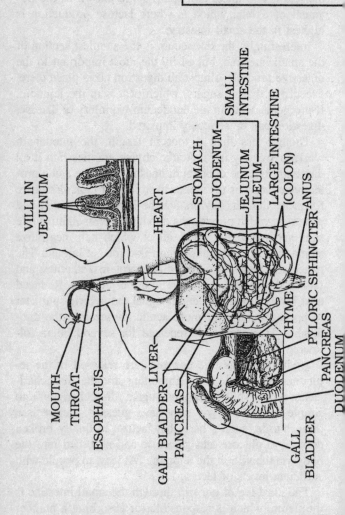

Anatomy of the digestive system.

VILLI IN JEJUNUM

HEART

STOMACH

DUODENUM

JEJUNUM

ILEUM

SMALL INTESTINE

LARGE INTESTINE (COLON)

ANUS

CHYME

PYLORIC SPHINCTER

PANCREAS

DUODENUM

GALL BLADDER

MOUTH

THROAT

ESOPHAGUS

LIVER

GALL BLADDER

PANCREAS

vitamins. Once food has reached this point, the small intestine has absorbed so much that our meal has been reduced to just a fraction of what it was when consumed. The remaining sluice is then pushed into the large intestine, more commonly known as the colon, for one last round of digestion and nutrient processing. The colon's most important job, however, is to absorb as much of the water it receives from the small intestine as possible, leaving just enough to keep our stools soft and mushy for painless elimination (constipation and hard, rocklike stools are often a sign of dehydration or a decrease in colonic transit function). The absorption of this water allows the body to take advantage of any remaining vitamins and other nutrients that may be left over—proof that digestion is, indeed, a very efficient process.

What's left after most of the water has been absorbed is waste matter, which is pushed into the rectum, where it sits until expelled via the anus. Feces is made up primarily of stuff that simply couldn't be digested, such as certain types of fibers, mucus, and other substances. It also contains a huge amount of bacteria, which are essential to proper digestion but can cause serious illness if accidentally consumed. (Recent reports of *E. coli* infections as a result of eating bacteria-tainted meat are good examples of this). As noted earlier, these same colonic bacteria feast on whatever lactose isn't absorbed by the intestines, producing their own lactase to split the complex sugar into its component parts, and sugar is fermented by bacteria, expelling large amounts of gas in the process. The result: many of the painful symptoms commonly associated with lactose intolerance, including bloating and diarrhea.

Q: Once the bacteria in the colon break down lactose into simple sugars, are these nutrients finally absorbed into the body?

A: No. Unlike the jejunum, the colon is not designed to absorb simple sugars such as glucose and galactose. So the sugars stay in the colon and provide additional food for the billions of bacteria there, which turn them into compounds known as short-chain fatty acids. This stimulates further intestinal function, known medically as peristalsis, and causes more unwanted water to be transported from the small intestine into the colon. In addition, the difference in concentration of water in the mucosa (mucous membrane) of the intestine and the intestinal cavity (the lumen) causes water to be secreted from the mucosa into the cavity. The gases produced by bacterial metabolization (primarily carbon dioxide, hydrogen and, sometimes, methane) and the rush of water combine to create many of the aggravating symptoms discussed above.

Q: I'm 40 years old and was recently diagnosed with moderate lactose intolerance. Since my health is important to me, I'm trying to learn as much about this condition as I can. Let's start at the beginning: what are the most common forms of lactose intolerance?

A: According to researchers, lactose intolerance can be divided into three different categories. Primary acquired lactose intolerance, which is genetic in origin and generally worsens over time, is by far the most common form of the condition. Though few accurate statistics are available, it would be safe to assume that 80 percent or more of lactose-intolerance cases are the result of primary acquired lactose intolerance. Secondary lactose intolerance, which is less common, typically results from situations that adversely affect the large intestine, such as infection, disease, surgery, or the use of certain medications. The rarest form of lactose intolerance is known as congenital lactose intolerance, a genetic defect that causes a baby to be born without the ability to digest lactose or many other naturally occurring sugars.

Q: How soon after birth does primary acquired lactose intolerance begin? When does the body begin to slow production of lactase?
A: The production of lactase and its eventual decline is an intriguing physiological phenomenon. Researchers have found that an 8-month-old fetus may have only 70 percent of the lactase activity it will have at birth. But as birth rapidly approaches, lactase production increases dramatically as the baby's body prepares it for a high-milk diet.

As noted in Chapter One, a baby's ability to digest milk peaks within days of birth and begins a slow descent from then on. Lactase levels are usually high during the first weeks following birth because mother's milk or cow's milk-based formula is the primary source of nutrition for most infants, and without lactase they would literally starve to death. However, as soon as solid, non–milk based foods are introduced, lactase levels begin to decline—a natural situation that cannot be reversed. By the time an infant is on solid foods, its lactase production has slowed dramatically (remember, it's the rare individual who does not produce any lactase at all). In most people, lactase levels continue to decline gradually as they age, until the body simply cannot handle large amounts of lactose anymore and symptoms begin to appear.

Q: How does the body know when to slow lactase production?

A: In most cases, the reduction in lactase production is a genetically programmed, spontaneous occurrence. It's as if the body suddenly flips its "lactase production" switch from on to off. Of course, in most cases this is a gradual reduction, and the intestines will continue to produce small amounts of the enzyme for most of our lives. If it didn't, we wouldn't be able to consume any lactose at all.

Lactase deficiency happens at different times for different people. There is no set age for lactase production to slow. In many cases it occurs around age 2 or 3, though in some individuals it may not occur until age 6 or later. In the vast majority of people prone to lactose intolerance, lactase deficiency has occurred by the onset of puberty, and lactase production will continue to slowly diminish for many years to come. Because everyone is unique, some people find themselves unable to consume normal amounts of lactose at a very early age, while others continue to enjoy dairy products well into adulthood. And many will never suffer from lactose intolerance at all.

Q: Can anything be done to stimulate lactase production or maintain current lactase levels in people with primary acquired lactase intolerance?

A: At this time, no. The rate of lactase production is genetically programmed, and nothing can alter that. As mentioned in Chapter One, researchers working with lactose-intolerant rats were able to stimulate lactase production through gene therapy, but that currently is not an option for people with the condition.

Some people believe that consuming large amounts of

dairy products or taking lactase supplements will stimulate production of the enzyme, but the body doesn't work like that. Consuming large amounts of dairy products will only result in painful symptoms in most individuals with lactose intolerance, and lactase supplements only help you digest lactose at the time they are taken. They have no long-term effects.

Q: A friend of mine told me that she became lactose intolerant as a result of intestinal surgery. Is this an example of secondary lactose intolerance as mentioned earlier?

A: Yes. Any form of lactose intolerance without a genetic influence is called secondary lactose intolerance, and your friend's condition is an excellent example.

Indeed, secondary lactose intolerance is a relatively common condition and can result from a wide array of situations and diseases. For example, the majority of people with untreated celiac disease (a condition resulting from a sensitivity to gluten, a protein found in wheat and other grains) also suffer from related lactose intolerance. So do nearly half of the people diagnosed each year with various inflammatory bowel diseases, such as Crohn's disease. Parasites of the small intestine, including giardia, dysentery, and hookworm, can also cause lactose intolerance by interfering with the intestine's ability to produce lactase. And so can intestinal surgery, as your friend's case so clearly illustrates.

Secondary lactose intolerance can also result from a pancreatic insufficiency caused by such things as cystic fibrosis or excessive alcohol consumption, as well as the use of certain antibiotics and cancer drugs. Malnutrition in its many forms—a very common problem worldwide—is another frequent cause of the condition.

Q: How do all of these things affect the intestines to reduce or inhibit the production of lactase?

A: In the majority of cases, the disease or condition affects the lactase-producing cells that line the small intestine, either shortening the life of such cells or adversely affecting their function. In a smaller number of cases, lactose intolerance results from the insufficient exposure of food to these lactase-producing cells. In other words, food races through the intestinal tract too quickly for the lactase to break down lactose. This most commonly occurs as a result of dumping syndrome from ulcer surgery, or following the removal of a section of diseased intestine (a procedure known medically as a resection) or intestinal bypass, a last-ditch treatment for morbid obesity that is rarely performed anymore.

Q: Of all of the conditions mentioned above, which one most commonly causes secondary lactose intolerance?

A: According to gastroenterologists, the most common cause of secondary lactose intolerance is severe infectious diarrhea. This can be caused by a wide range of organisms, including bacteria, viruses, and protozoa, all of which can wreak havoc on the human digestive system by damaging the intestinal lining. Such disorders can be extremely problematic, resulting in fever, nausea, diarrhea, headache, and fatigue, and may take a while to eliminate. In a frustrating turn of events, many sufferers recover from those miserable symptoms, only to find themselves afflicted with lactose intolerance. And the problem usually grows worse following additional infections or as an individual ages.

Q: Is secondary lactose intolerance resulting from infectious diarrhea more common in certain groups than others?

A: People who live in tropical regions where infectious bacteria and protozoa are common run a higher risk than other populations simply because their exposure to infectious agents tends to be greater. Exposure is less in the United States because we tend to practice greater health precautions than other regions in the world, but infectious diarrhea is still a concern. Young children are especially prone to such disorders because their immune systems are still developing, they tend to play in areas easily contaminated by animals, and they tend to put everything they find in their mouths. Gastroenterologists note that children under three years are so susceptible to infectious diarrhea that secondary lactose intolerance is far more prevalent than primary lactose intolerance in that population.

Q: Is secondary lactose intolerance a lifelong condition like primary acquired lactose intolerance, or is there a chance it'll go away?

A: It depends on the cause. Secondary lactose intolerance caused by certain diseases or medical procedures, such as intestinal surgery, is usually a lifelong condition. However, there are exceptions. For example, lactose intolerance caused by less serious diseases or the use of certain drugs may gradually clear up once the disease is cured or the drugs are discontinued. If you believe you have become lactose intolerant as a result of the medication you are taking, ask your doctor to perform a lactose-intolerance test. (See Chapter Three.) If the condition is confirmed, your doctor may be able to suggest alternative medications that aren't quite as hard on your digestive tract.

"I found that I had become mildly lactose intolerant as a result of the antibiotics I was taking for a stubborn stomach infection," notes Connie, a 38-year-old computer consultant. "I took the medication religiously on the advice of my doctor, and suddenly found myself suffering from embarrassing gas and intestinal rumbling anytime I ate more than moderate amounts of dairy products. This was frustrating because I love milk and other dairy foods, and I didn't want to have to cut back on my consumption. My doctor said that my condition was most likely caused by the antibiotics I was taking, and that it might be only temporary, though he could give me no guarantees. Thankfully, he was right. About six weeks after I stopped taking the antibiotics, I noticed that my tolerance for lactose seemed to be increasing. It never returned to what it was before I started taking my medication, but I'm able to enjoy almost all of my favorite foods without too much of a problem."

Q: Can anything be done to help the intestines recover from disease- or drug-related lactose intolerance?
A: If you are sure that your lactose intolerance is the result of a minor illness or a specific medication, you can often help your intestines recover and begin producing lactase again by following a very low-lactose diet for about a month or so afterward. A reduced workload allows your intestines to heal faster. After that, lactose levels should be increased gradually.

Q: My brother was recently diagnosed as having celiac disease. You mentioned this as a possible cause of secondary lactose intolerance. Could you give us

some additional information on this specific condition?

A: Celiac disease is a relatively common digestive disorder characterized by a sensitivity or intolerance to gluten, a protein found in grains such as wheat, rye, oats, and barley. It afflicts an estimated 1 in 2,500 people, and goes by a number of other names, including gluten-induced enteropathy, gluten intolerance, celiac sprue, and nontropical sprue.

For most people, gluten is a good source of important nutrients. It consists of water-insoluble glutenin and soluble gliadins. However, gliadins are toxic and in sensitive individuals can damage the intestinal lining, known as the mucosa, making the absorption of nutrients difficult and sometimes resulting in concomitant (associated) lactose intolerance.

Celiac disease is a strange condition, and researchers are still unsure why it occurs. Symptoms are many and can include diarrhea or constipation, gas, weight loss, abdominal bloating, fatigue, greasy stool, and unexplained increase in appetite. Serious cases of celiac disease can result in iron-deficiency anemia or osteomalacia, a disorder of the bones caused by vitamin D deficiency. It has been shown that when gluten is injected into the ileum of celiac disease patients, tissue changes begin to occur within hours.

Q: Are certain populations more at risk of celiac disease than others?

A: Yes. According to gastroenterologists, up to 70 percent of celiac disease sufferers are female, though researchers aren't sure why the disorder afflicts women so much more than men. It also occurs more frequently in people of northwestern European ancestry. In fact, the highest incidence of celiac disease in the world is in Galway, Ireland, where 1 in every 300 people are afflicted. Those least likely to develop celiac disease are individuals of African, Asian, Jewish, and Mediterranean descent—oddly, the groups most likely to be lactose intolerant.

Researchers suspect a genetic predisposition because the incidence of the disease is far more common among siblings than in the general population.

Q: Can celiac disease be cured?
A: No. Like lactose intolerance, it can only be controlled through diet management. This means the elimination of all foods containing gluten—a chore almost as difficult as avoiding lactose. Wheat flour is a very common ingredient in foods ranging from salad dressings, instant coffee, and canned foods to candy bars and popular condiments, including catsup and mustard. As a result, people with a gluten intolerance must carefully monitor the ingredients of the foods they eat at home and in restaurants.

Luckily, there are a number of safe alternatives to wheat. Flours made from rice, soybean, buckwheat, potato, and corn can all be digested by individuals with celiac disease and can be substituted for wheat flour in many recipes. There are a number of cookbooks for people who cannot tolerate gluten in their diets. Two volumes recommended by dieticians are *Gourmet Food on a Wheat-Free Diet* and *Easy Rice Flour Recipes*, both by Marion Wood.

Q: In addition to celiac disease, what other intestinal diseases can cause secondary lactose intolerance?
A: There are a lot of them, though doctors note that the

incidence of lactose intolerance related to these disorders is actually pretty small. Small bowel diseases, such as Crohn's disease, can cause secondary lactose intolerance. Large bowel diseases, such as irritable bowel syndrome (also known as irritable colon, spastic colon, and mucous colitis), diverticulitis, diverticulosis, and ulcerative colitis, can mimic lactose intolerance but do not cause secondary lactose intolerance. As mentioned earlier, the most common causes of secondary lactose intolerance are infectious—viral, bacterial, and protozoal—or due to medication use. In tropical areas the most common infectious causes are tropical sprue and parasitic protozoa. Conditions that actually cause lactose intolerance do so by damaging the intestinal lining. We'll discuss many of these disorders in greater detail in Chapter Five.

Q: My uncle was a hard drinker all his life, but managed to save himself through Alcoholics Anonymous. One of the leftover results of his alcoholism, according to his doctor, is lactose intolerance. I don't understand the connection.

A: It's simple—your uncle's years of drinking physically damaged his intestines to the point where lactose could no longer be digested properly. Chronic alcohol abuse can cause lactose intolerance in several ways, including through malnutrition, pancreatic insufficiency, and possibly through local damage to the intestine.

The intestines, for all their hard work and the efficiency with which they do it, are actually quite sensitive and fragile. Any abuse or physical damage can result in reduced lactase production and/or lactose malabsorption. Sometimes this condition is temporary and sometimes, as in your uncle's case, it's permanent.

Many people who undergo intestinal surgery for whatever reason find that they suddenly cannot tolerate dairy products the way they used to. This is especially true if a section of the jejunum is involved because that's where lactase activity is strongest, but it can also occur if any major section of the intestinal tract is removed. The intestinal villi are very sensitive and easily sent into a temporary dysfunctional state. In most cases they eventually recover and lactose digestion returns to normal. But, again, sometimes it doesn't. Not surprisingly, most cases of lactose intolerance resulting from surgery on the jejunum are permanent.

Individuals who experience postoperative lactose intolerance should notify their doctors because a lactose-free diet may be necessary to give the intestines time to recover. This is also true of those afflicted with secondary lactose intolerance resulting from other causes.

Q: Can a blow to the lower abdomen, such as a hard hit during football, cause secondary lactose intolerance?
A: In theory, yes, although secondary lactose intolerance resulting from such an injury would most likely be a temporary and reversible condition, unless there was massive trauma to the bowel that required a bowel resection. Remember: Any damage to the intestines can send them into shock, reducing lactase production and thus lactose digestion. For this reason we should always use common sense in protecting ourselves from injury— especially our chest and abdominal region. Seat belts, for example, should always be worn when driving to prevent a potentially damaging collision with the steering wheel in case of an accident. And protective gear should always be worn when playing contact sports such

as football. You can't be too careful when it comes to your body.

Q: I've been reading a lot lately about the occurrence, prevention, and treatment of colon cancer. Can colon cancer also result in lactose intolerance?
A: There is no explicit relationship between colon cancer and lactose intolerance. However, common treatments for colon cancer such as surgery, radiation, and chemotherapy may adversely affect the intestines' ability to produce lactase, resulting in the condition.

By the way, colorectal cancer is quite common, so everyone should be aware of its symptoms and see their doctor at the first indication of a possible tumor. The disease has a high cure rate if detected early.

Q: Two of my dearest friends were recently diagnosed with colon cancer, so I know how insidious this disease can be. Thankfully, both cases were detected early and both of my friends are expected to recover fully. Could you please give us a little more information about this all-too-common disease, including rate of incidence and risk factors?
A: According to cancer experts, colorectal cancer is second only to lung cancer as a cause of cancer death in the United States. More than 150,000 new cases are diagnosed and approximately 50,000 people die from the disease each year. Colorectal cancer is seen most commonly in upper-socioeconomic populations living in urban areas.

There are a number of risk factors for colorectal cancer, the biggest being diet and family history. Epidemiologic studies in the United States and abroad have found a fairly strong link between colorectal cancer deaths and the traditional Western diet, which is high in calories, meat protein, and dietary fats and oils. Not surprisingly, those populations whose lifestyles and eating habits tend to be more healthful, such as Mormons and Seventh Day Adventists, have significantly lower rates of colorectal cancer than others. And those countries that have adopted the traditional American diet, such as Japan, are seeing increased rates of colorectal cancer in their populations.

Researchers also believe that there can be a genetic component in the development of certain kinds of colorectal cancer. In almost all cases of colorectal cancer, there is a mutation in a gene called adenomatous polyposis coli (APC), which normally halts cell growth. When APC goes awry, however, it causes unchecked cell growth, or cancer. The APC gene has been identified in patients with a family history of colon polyps (growths in the lining of the colon), a condition called familial adenomatous polyposis (FAP). This condition leads to colon cancer if the colon is not removed. An estimated 25 percent of colorectal patients have a family history of the disease, which suggests a potential hereditary predisposition.

Certain kinds of bowel disorders, such as ulcerative colitis and Crohn's disease, may also play a role in the development of various types of colorectal cancer, doctors add. Studies show that the risk of colorectal cancer in a patient with inflammatory bowel disease is fairly small during the first 10 years of the disease, but then appears to increase by up to 1.0 percent a year. (See Chapter Five for more information on inflammatory bowel disease and related conditions.)

Q: What are the most common symptoms of colorectal cancer?

A: They depend on the location of the tumor within the colon. In general, though, early signs of potential colorectal cancer include sudden changes in bowel habits, such as persistent constipation or diarrhea, and blood in the stool. However, it must be noted that blood in the stool may not be readily evident (doctors refer to this as "occult") and can be detected only through a laboratory test on a stool sample. Don't rely on commercially available home occult-blood tests. They may be convenient, but some cancer experts feel they're not accurate enough to be trusted.

Symptoms of more advanced colorectal cancer may include abdominal cramps or the feeling that your bowels are always full, gradual weight loss and accompanying loss of appetite, and anemia (commonly characterized by general fatigue, weakness, and stools that are black or bloodred).

Q: How is colorectal cancer typically treated?
A: The complete surgical removal of the tumor or tumors typically offers the best prognosis. During surgery, the surgeon usually checks the other organs in the abdominal cavity to make sure the cancer has not spread. Radiation therapy is often recommended for patients with rectal cancer because there is a 30 to 40 percent probability of recurrence in that region following complete surgical removal of cancerous growths. This high rate of recurrence is believed to be due to the fact that the tight space within the pelvis limits the extent of the surgery and because the rich lymphatic network of the pelvic sidewall next to the rectum encourages the spread of tumor cells into nearby tissue.

A combination of surgery, radiation therapy, and/or chemotherapy is often used to treat patients with advanced-stage colorectal cancers to eliminate undetectable microtumors in other areas of the body and to increase the probability of a full recovery.

Q: Colorectal cancer sounds serious. What can I do to prevent the onset of this potentially deadly disease?

A: Colorectal cancer is serious, but there are steps you can take to prevent it from developing. Because there is an apparent link between diet and colorectal cancer, most experts recommend a diet that is low in saturated fats and high in fiber and complex carbohydrates. Dietary fat is an especially important issue because studies show that it can increase bile acids in the colon which in turn promote the development and growth of colon tumors, so do what you can to cut down. In one British study, researchers compared the dietary histories of 50 colorectal-cancer patients with those of a closely matched, healthy control group and found that the cancer patients consumed an average of 14 percent more calories (mostly in the form of fat and carbohydrates) than those who did not have cancer.

It also apparently helps to add more calcium and vitamin D to your diet (something you should be doing anyway if you have lactose intolerance). In one 20-year study, it was found that men who consumed the least milk had almost three times the risk of getting colorectal cancer as those who drank the most. The reason is unclear, though some researchers speculate that calcium, aided by vitamin D, combines with bile acids and fatty acids in the colon to form insoluble calcium compounds, which are flushed out of the body. Of course, people with lactose intolerance often cannot consume milk or other calcium-rich dairy foods, but there are plenty of nondairy alternatives, including leafy green vegetables and dietary supplements.

Regular exercise is also vitally important in preventing colorectal cancer—especially if you have a relatively sedentary job and lifestyle. Researchers at the University of Southern California School of Medicine looked at the lifestyles of nearly 3,000 male colon-cancer patients and found that those with sedentary jobs (meaning they sat all day) such as accounting and law were at almost 60 percent higher risk for colorectal cancer than men with more active occupations, such as mail carrier. Men with moderately active jobs, such as truck driver or salesman, had a rate of colon cancer approximately halfway between the two.

The amount of exercise you do doesn't have to be extreme—just performed regularly. A brisk walk around the block, a couple of games of tennis, or a few laps on the pool three or four times a week should be sufficient, but the more the better. If you find it difficult to get motivated, join a gym or fitness center. Or better yet, find an "exercise buddy," someone you can count on to exercise with you. Most people find exercise easier when they have someone to talk to and keep them company.

"Both my father and my uncle developed colorectal cancer, and my uncle died from the disease, so I'm especially cautious," says Ray, a 38-year-old electrical engineer. "I get a physical exam once a year that includes a digital exam for prostate and rectal tumors and an occult-blood test. The digital exam isn't fun, but I know it's important so I grit my teeth and get it over with. I also try to watch my diet by eating plenty of fresh fruits, vegetables, and fiber-rich whole-grain breads. I'm not a fanatic about my food—I like hamburger and steak as much as the next guy—but I do eat a lot more poultry and fish than beef. I also exercise by running a couple of miles every day after work. Not only does it help keep colon cancer at bay, but it's also good for my heart and lungs.

"I may still develop colon cancer despite what I do because of my family history, but I'm going to fight it every step of the way. And because I get an annual physical exam, I know that if I do develop the disease, my doctor will catch it in the early stages. Colon cancer isn't something you should dwell on, but it's certainly something you should think about."

Q: Earlier you mentioned a third type of lactose intolerance called congenital lactose intolerance. Could you please discuss this condition a bit more?
A: Congenital lactose intolerance is the rarest form of the condition and occurs in babies born with a genetic defect that results in the inability to produce any lactase at all. This, in turn, results in a complete inability to digest lactose or any other common sugars, including sucrose and fructose. In the old days, congenital lactose intolerance was almost always fatal because babies were unable to digest their mother's milk and subsequently starved to death. Today, congenital lactose intolerance can be identified almost immediately after birth, and babies born with the condition usually thrive on soy-based or other sugar-free formulas.

Lactose intolerance resulting from low lactase production (not to be confused with congenital lactose intolerance) often occurs in premature babies, and doctors are starting to see more of it thanks to advances in the technology used to keep preemies alive. A higher occurrence of lactose intolerance in preemies makes sense because, as noted earlier, lactase is one of the last digestive enzymes a fetus manufactures prior to birth.

However, not all premature babies develop the condition. Many are able to tolerate milk (breast milk, or milk-based formulas) well (though there is a big difference between lactose tolerance and lactose absorption. Just because a baby is able to tolerate milk doesn't necessarily mean it's getting all the nutrients it should from it). According to researchers, there are a number of reasons for this. Perhaps most importantly, the first feedings a premature infant receives apparently helps to stimulate the production of lactase in its intestines. In addition, the milk produced by a new mother in the first few feedings following birth contains lower levels of lactose than the milk she will produce later on. A third factor is a premature baby's digestive tract. It's almost sterile at birth, having yet to be exposed to the various bacteria that will eventually take up residence there. And as we know, bacteria are one of the major contributors to the symptoms of lactose intolerance.

THREE

How is Lactose
Intolerance Diagnosed?

IT SEEMED THAT ANDY HAD ALWAYS SUFFERED FROM what his mother called a nervous stomach. As a child, he experienced frequent bouts of intestinal bloating, cramps, and diarrhea, and missed many days of school because of it. The symptoms were particularly problematic because they usually occurred without warning and for no apparent reason. One moment Andy would be feeling fine, the next he would be doubled over with searing intestinal cramps that would inevitably result in a race to the bathroom. As the problem grew increasingly common, Andy came to dread traveling even short distances from home for fear that he would suddenly be stricken with explosive diarrhea. Family vacations, once the highlight of his summer break, became stressful events that were seldom pleasant or fun.

Concerned about the growing frequency of Andy's intestinal troubles, his parents turned to the boy's longtime pediatrician for advice and comfort. The doctor nodded thoughtfully as 11-year-old Andy described his symptoms, then listened to Andy's heart, checked his ears, and immediately diagnosed Andy's problem as ''an irritable bowel.'' There was little that could be done about it, the doctor added, though a bland diet and a reduction in stress might help. It was just something Andy would have to live with until he grew out of it.

. But Andy didn't grow out of it. He continued to experience severe digestive distress through high school, though the problem lessened somewhat when he went off to college. Even then, however, Andy lived in constant fear of its onset, and found his social life suffering as a result. It took all the resolve he could muster to ask a girl out on a date, though he usually enjoyed himself when he did. Luckily, most of the girls whom he dated were understanding when his digestive difficulties put a sudden crimp in their plans.

Andy married shortly after college and took a job as an architect with a large New York firm. He was good at his job and a popular employee. He managed to keep his digestive problems a secret until one day, in the middle of an important meeting, he was suddenly afflicted with gas, bloating, and intestinal pressure. Apologizing profusely, Andy raced from the room and into the nearest toilet, where he silently cursed his ''irritable bowel.''

That night, Andy discussed the embarrassing incident with his wife, Kathryn, who in turn mentioned it to her sister, Cheryl, a pediatric nurse. Cheryl commented that the childhood diagnosis of ''irritable bowel'' didn't sound right and suggested Andy see a gastroenterologist for a more comprehensive workup. Kathryn mentioned Cheryl's concerns to Andy, who reluctantly agreed.

Two days later, Andy met with a well-known gastroenterologist, who took a full medical history and talked with Andy at length about his recurring problem. He asked Andy if the symptoms seemed to occur at specific times, such as after meals—especially meals heavy in dairy products. Suddenly a lightbulb went off over Andy's head. "I had never realized it before, but that's exactly how things usually worked," Andy recalled recently. "Certain foods triggered symptoms, but others did not. But it wasn't until I talked with the gastroenterologist that I realized my problems occurred more frequently after eating certain dairy products. The morning of my embarrassing sprint from the meeting, for example, I had consumed a large glass of milk with my cereal and fruit. Two hours later, all hell broke loose."

The gastroenterologist told Andy that his problem sounded like lactose intolerance, and suggested something called a "breath hydrogen test" to confirm it. Andy immediately agreed. The test, which involved drinking a mixture of lactose and water and blowing into a series of special bags, was performed, and the breath samples were sent to a lab for analysis. The results confirmed the gastroenterologist's initial diagnosis of lactose intolerance. All of the problems Andy had experienced throughout his life were the result of a natural inability to digest milk sugar properly.

"I'm managing my condition very well on a low-lactose diet, and my gastrointestinal problems have decreased more than 90 percent as a result," Andy notes. "I can't really be mad at my pediatrician for misdiagnosing my condition when I was 11 because back then they just didn't know that much about lactose intolerance, especially doctors outside of gastroenterology. But I was foolish for not seeking help sooner once I had grown up. Recurrent gastric distress isn't something you have to live with. Whatever the cause, it can almost certainly be diagnosed and treated. That's a lesson I learned the hard way.''

Indeed, lactose intolerance is very easy to diagnose and manage. In this chapter, we'll discuss the various types of tests currently available, the role of the primary care physician and the gastroenterologist in the diagnosis and management of lactose intolerance, and how to tell the difference between lactose intolerance and milk allergy.

Q: I've been experiencing increasingly frequent digestive problems that are indicative of lactose intolerance and realized it was time I finally saw a doctor about it. Must I see a gastroenterologist or can my primary care physician do the job?

A: Your primary care physician should be able to help you. It used to be that physicians outside of gastroenterology (the specialty concerned with disorders of the digestive system) weren't as familiar with the symptoms, high incidence, or diagnosis of lactose intolerance, but that has changed in recent years as the condition receives more and more publicity in the medical journals as well as in the general press.

Since you already suspect that your symptoms may be caused by poor lactose digestion, make your concerns known to your primary care physician. But don't expect him to agree instantly and send you on your way. No physician worth his medical degree would make a diagnosis based only on a patient's assumptions. Your doctor will most likely take a full medical history and then give you a complete physical examination to rule out any obvious organic causes of your symptoms, such as colon cancer or Crohn's disease. If you appear to be in otherwise good health and your symptoms truly seem to indicate that you're suffering from lactose intolerance, your physician will probably then suggest one or more tests for an accurate diagnosis. If the tests are positive, your primary care physician can then work with you to develop a diet plan that will help keep your symptoms under control.

Q: I'm sure my primary care physician is competent. But wouldn't it be easier just to go to a gastroenterologist first? After all, they specialize in these kinds of things.

A: There are a number of very good reasons why your initial consultation should be with your primary care physician. First of all, he probably knows you and your health better than anyone else. If your primary care physician has been your doctor for a while, he's well aware of your general health, any medical problems you've had in the past, your family medical history and what medications you're currently taking. In short, he knows you and your body inside and out. That's what makes your primary care physician your most effective first line of defense when it comes to your health.

Gastroenterologists specialize in digestive disorders, but unless your case is particularly complicated, you probably don't need that level of expertise. Most general practitioners are well aware of the prevalence of lactose intolerance, as well as its diagnosis and management, and in most cases they're fully competent to address this particular medical condition.

Another good reason to see your primary care physician first is cost. In general, a visit to a specialist such as a gastroenterologist will always cost you more than a visit to a general practitioner because you're paying for the specialist's additional training, knowledge, and expertise. That's great if you have a serious or very complicated gastrointestinal ailment, but most cases of lactose intolerance are neither serious nor complicated. So why pay for an expensive specialist when you can get the same results from a doctor who is familiar with you and your health at a fraction of the cost?

Of course, that's not to suggest that gastroenterologists do not play an important role in the diagnosis and management of lactose intolerance and related ailments—they most certainly do. Anything related to the human gastrointestinal system falls under the purview of gastroenterology, and much of the research into lactose intolerance has been performed by gastroenterologists eager to help those who suffer from this common and discomforting condition. But for the average lactose-intolerant patient, it's probably best to save a visit to the gastroenterologist for something more serious.

A third reason for seeing your primary care physician first is because you may have to. Many HMOs and other third-party health care providers require clients to see their primary care physician before they see a specialist. This is to prevent clients from seeking out more expensive treatment when their primary care physician can treat them just as easily. Of course, many emergency situations are exempt from this rule, but a suspicion of lactose intolerance is hardly an emergency. If your situation proves to be more complicated than your primary care provider can safely handle, he may then make a referral to a gastroenterologist. However, most HMOs will not let you see just any gastroenterologist—this doctor, too, must be someone on your plan. For further information on this particular issue, read the literature provided by your HMO or call to find out if and how you are covered.

Q: I recently saw my doctor about recurrent gas and diarrhea following meals, and he immediately diagnosed my condition as lactose intolerance. However, he didn't perform any diagnostic tests, and that has me concerned. Shouldn't he have done at least one test, just to be sure?

A: Absolutely. The fact that your doctor diagnosed your health problem as lactose intolerance without conducting a single test suggests he really doesn't know that much about the condition. If he did, he would realize that many problems can mimic its symptoms and that a lactose-intolerance test is essential for an accurate diagnosis.

It could simply be that your doctor felt a lactose-intolerance test was unnecessary based on your specific symptoms. But regardless of the reason, he is jeopardizing your health.

If you really like your doctor and this is the first problem you've had with him, bring up the issue of testing during your next visit and tell him you would like to take a breath hydrogen test or other exam to confirm his diagnosis. If he has your best interests at heart, he'll agree. If he tries to talk you out of it, seek a second opinion.

Q: Under what conditions might my primary care physician refer me to a gastroenterologist?

A: There are a number of reasons. One of the most obvious would be if your symptoms indicate lactose intolerance but your tests come back negative for that specific condition. If your doctor is unable to explain your specific symptoms adequately, he might refer you to a gastroenterologist with greater experience in that particular field. Any indication of a serious gastrointestinal problem, such as colon cancer, would also be sufficient grounds for a referral to a gastroenterologist.

A referral to a specialist such as a gastroenterologist is usually made when a general practitioner or family physician concludes that his patient needs more expert care than he can provide. It doesn't necessarily mean that there is anything seriously wrong with you, only that your primary care physician is erring on the side of caution in having you checked out by someone with greater expertise. If such a referral is made, make sure you ask your primary care doctor why he feels it's necessary and what you should expect.

Q: What information should I give my primary care physician when I see her for suspected lactose intolerance? And what kinds of questions should I ask?

A: Let's start with the questions. The most important one, obviously, is how much expertise does she have in diagnosing and managing lactose intolerance and related disorders? Most general practitioners have a fair amount of knowledge and experience, but some may not because of the nature and/or location of their practice. If your doctor has had little expertise in this specific area, ask if she can refer you to someone who is more knowledgeable.

Another important question to pose to your doctor is her philosophy on lactose intolerance. Some doctors believe the condition is extremely common, others believe it's just media hype. If your doctor believes that lactose intolerance isn't nearly as common as others believe it to be, she may not take you or your symptoms seriously, or she may assume it's all in your head. Your doctor's philosophy will affect how she views your condition as well as methods of diagnosis, so make sure you're in agreement on this.

You should also ask your doctor what types of tests she uses to diagnose suspected lactose intolerance, how much such tests will cost, how long it will take to get the results back (most doctors send the tests to an outside lab for analysis), whether the tests are covered by your insurance, what she will suggest if your tests are negative (meaning you are not lactose intolerant), and whether she will be able to help you develop an effective dietary-management regimen if they are positive.

As for information, the best thing you can do is provide your doctor with as much information about your condition as you can. This includes what your symptoms are, their intensity, when symptoms first became noticeable, whether you had symptoms as a child, when they most frequently occur (such as after specific meals), what you have done in the past to alleviate your symptoms (such as the use of antacids and antigas and antidiarrhea medications), and whether they were at all effective. If you fear you'll forget something, don't hesitate to write it all down before your office visit.

Other information your doctor should be made aware of includes recent changes in diet, recent illnesses or accidents (especially those involving the abdominal region), recent increases in stress or anxiety levels, recent problems at home or at work, recent visits abroad (many parasitic illnesses can mimic the symptoms of lactose intolerance), and whether there is a family history of lactose intolerance or related problems. You should also tell your doctor if you are experiencing pain as a result of your symptoms, or have noticed blood in your stool. Having all of this information and anything else you can think of handy when you visit your doctor will help make the accurate diagnosis of your problem easier and quicker.

Remember: The diagnosis and treatment of any health problems you may have, including lactose intolerance, should be a collaborative effort between you and your doctor. It's unfair and unrealistic to expect your doctor to do all the work, though that's the mind-set of most Americans. Your physician may be able to diagnose your problem and suggest helpful management techniques, but it's your responsibility to put those suggestions into action.

Q: My doctor said she would have to do something called a "differential diagnosis" to accurately confirm my self-diagnosis of lactose intolerance. What's a differential diagnosis? Should I be concerned?

A: Relax, you have nothing to worry about. A differential diagnosis is merely the act of sifting through all possible answers to a problem until only the correct one remains. It's a standard procedure in medicine and doctors do it all the time.

No doubt your self-diagnosis of lactose intolerance was based on your symptoms. It may seem open and shut to you, but probably less so to your doctor. Your symptoms may suggest lactose intolerance, but they could also be indicative of other gastrointestinal disorders. Just to be safe, your doctor will take all possible answers into consideration and methodically discard them until she has narrowed your problem down to the most probable. It's a lot like being Sherlock Holmes and analyzing all of the clues. If, as you suspect, the culprit ultimately appears to be lactose intolerance, your doctor will likely prescribe one or more tests for the condition to make absolutely sure.

The differential diagnosis is important in medicine because many disorders mimic others, and lactose intolerance is one of the most mimicked of all. Just because your symptoms seem to indicate lactose intolerance doesn't necessarily mean you really have the condition. Listen to your physician and do what she recommends.

Q: If tests show that my symptoms aren't caused by lactose intolerance, what else could it be?
A: Almost anything. As noted earlier, a wide range of disorders mimic the symptoms of lactose intolerance, including certain inflammatory bowel diseases, irritable bowel syndrome, and colon cancer, all of which will be discussed in greater detail in Chapter Five: Diseases That Mimic Lactose Intolerance. Intestinal distress can also be triggered by a number of lifestyle factors, including stress and anxiety, excessive alcohol consumption, and the use of certain drugs. Even something as innocuous as spicy foods can cause gas, bloating, and diarrhea in sensitive individuals. Once your doctor has ruled out lactose intolerance, he can concentrate on other potential causes.

Q: After years of suffering from what seems to be lactose intolerance, I'm finally ready to have my condition checked out. What are the most common tests used to confirm lactose intolerance?
A: There are more than 15 distinct medical tests for the diagnosis of lactose intolerance, but by far the most commonly used is what's known as a breath hydrogen test (BHT). This test is based on the fact that hydrogen gas is rarely found in the human body. It is not produced by

any natural bodily functions and is almost nonexistent in our breath when we exhale. That is, of course, unless we are lactose intolerant. Researchers have found that hydrogen is produced in abundance by intestinal bacteria as it ferments undigested lactose. Quite a bit of this hydrogen gas passes through the intestinal wall and into the bloodstream, where it is carried to the lungs and expelled in the breath. This is fortunate, because a hydrogen colon test would be much more difficult, not to mention extremely uncomfortable.

The hydrogen breath test is a very accurate diagnosis of lactose intolerance because the gas is normally so uncommon in the breath. In fact, a measurement of more than 20 parts per million of hydrogen in the air exhaled is usually accepted as proof that lactose is not being digested well in the intestines.

A hydrogen breath test is very easy and completely painless. It is usually performed in the morning following a 12-hour fast (meaning you can have no food or drink during that time period) and consists of blowing through a mouthpiece into a special bag at regular intervals. The first bag is what's known as a reference baseline. After that, you'll be asked to drink a solution of lactose and water, though an increasing number of doctors are turning to regular milk because it more accurately reflects the everyday consumption of lactose. The amount of lactose in the solution may vary from 10 to 50 grams. Higher levels help identify more lactose-intolerant people, but such levels can also cause greater intestinal distress in sensitive individuals.

Symptoms of lactose intolerance are rarely exhibited immediately. It takes a bit of time for the lactose to pass through the intestines and for bacterial fermentation to take place. You will likely be asked to blow into additional bags at intervals of 15 minutes or more, and for up to several hours. An extended period is often necessary because some people do not show symptoms for up to three hours or more after lactose consumption. A longer test session may also be required if your doctor uses milk instead of a lactose-and-water solution because milk solids can delay gastric emptying. Symptoms such as gas or bloating will be noted by the doctor, though they are not necessarily strong indicators of lactose intolerance by themselves.

Few doctors can analyze breath samples in their offices because the necessary equipment is extremely expensive. Most of the time, the samples are sent to an outside laboratory for analysis. The breath hydrogen test is extremely accurate, detecting levels as small as 2 parts per million, but it's the high reading that's important. A reading of more than 20 parts per million is pretty definitive proof of a lactose-digestion problem.

Q: I've heard of a new test called the methane breath test. Can you tell me about it?
A: The methane breath test is an up-and-coming diagnostic test that is not yet available. Its purpose is to analyze breath samples for methane, which is produced by bacteria in the colon different from those that produce hydrogen. The methane-producing bacteria are unique in that they feed on the hydrogen and carbon dioxide produced by other bacteria as they ferment undigested lactose and other carbohydrates. Not all lactose-intolerant people will show methane in their breath, but those who do usually show a rise similar to that of breath hydrogen.

The discovery of methane in your breath, however, may be a sign of other gastrointestinal disorders, including Crohn's disease. Thus a positive methane test would need to be followed up with additional testing.

Q: What are the greatest benefits of the breath hydrogen test?

A: The breath hydrogen test is preferred by doctors and patients for a number of reasons. First of all, it's extremely easy to administer and is completely noninvasive (meaning you won't be stuck with needles or poked and prodded in uncomfortable places). The BHT is also relatively inexpensive compared to many other available tests, and the results are extremely accurate. As a result, it has pretty much become the standard for the diagnosis of lactose intolerance.

Q: I recently received a breath hydrogen test, and it confirmed that I was lactose intolerant. I was asked to drink a strong lactose mixture, and the resulting symptoms were much more severe than those I experience after drinking a glass of regular milk or eating a bowl of ice cream. Wouldn't the use of ordinary dairy products produce a more natural measurement?

A: You raise a very valid issue. As noted earlier, a growing number of doctors are performing breath hydrogen tests using ordinary milk instead of a mixture of lactose and water for exactly that reason—milk produces symptoms under natural, everyday conditions, and thus offers a more accurate indication of an individual's degree of lactose intolerance.

The lactose load consumed during a breath hydrogen test can be as high as 50 grams—the equivalent of drinking nearly a quart of milk in one sitting, and on an empty stomach. Worse, a solution of lactose and water doesn't provide the natural buffering offered by the solids found in regular milk, or by the foods that are typically consumed with milk at mealtime. These and other factors help people tolerate lactose a little better.

Some doctors like to perform breath hydrogen tests by the book, while others are willing to experiment a little. If you would prefer to consume milk rather than the traditional lactose-and-water solution, mention this to you doctor. If he balks, ask him why. He may have a very sound reason for wanting to stick with lactose and water.

Q: Is there a correlation between a high breath hydrogen reading and the severity of symptoms? In other words, are symptoms usually worse in people with very high breath hydrogen levels?
A: There is no apparent correlation between breath hydrogen levels and the severity of lactose-intolerance symptoms. Some individuals with levels just over 20 parts per million may suffer from severe symptoms, while others with much higher breath hydrogen levels may have only moderate symptoms. The important thing is that the test accurately reflects an inability to properly digest lactose.

Q: Can a breath hydrogen test reveal how much lactase is being produced by the intestines?
A: No. The test isn't designed to provide information like that. All it notes is the level of hydrogen in the breath you exhale.

Q: The breath hydrogen test sounds like the perfect tool for diagnosing lactose intolerance. Does it have any drawbacks?
A: The breath hydrogen test has pretty much become

the gold standard for the diagnosis of lactose intolerance, but it's not perfect. For example, it is not recommended for people taking antibiotics because the antibiotics can temporarily wipe out the bacteria that produce hydrogen, resulting in a false-negative result. Bacterial overgrowth (which can arise from conditions such as diabetes or from previous bowel operations, for example) can cause a false-positive result.

Another factor is whether your intestines are home to hydrogen-producing bacteria. Studies have found that up to 20 percent of the population have intestinal bacteria that cannot produce hydrogen. Obviously, this would result in a negative result despite the onset of telltale lactose-intolerance symptoms. Luckily, there are additional tests that can confirm the existence of non-hydrogen-producing bacteria, and your doctor will no doubt recommend one if the combination of a negative test result and obvious symptoms suggests the need. If you are one of the small minority of people who has these bacteria, you may need to use an alternative lactose-intolerance test.

Q: For a number of reasons, my doctor has suggested that I take a blood glucose test instead of a hydrogen breath test in an attempt to determine whether I really have lactose intolerance. What does this test entail?

A: Before the development of the breath hydrogen test, the blood glucose test was the test of choice among physicians for the diagnosis of lactose intolerance. In fact, it was so widely used that it was—and still is—commonly known as the lactose tolerance test (LTT). Today, however, it is usually used only in those rare cases when a breath hydrogen test is inappropriate, such as when lung disease or other medical conditions would make blowing into a bag difficult.

The blood glucose test, as its name implies, measures increases in blood glucose levels (if any) following lactose consumption. In a lactose-tolerant individual, lactose is easily digested and its component parts—glucose and galactose—are readily absorbed into the body, resulting in a noticeable elevation in blood glucose levels. But if an individual's lactase levels are low, lactose digestion is poor and there is little if any increase in blood glucose levels.

The blood glucose test is easy to administer. As with the hydrogen breath test, it is typically conducted in the morning on an empty stomach following a 12-hour fast. A baseline blood sample is drawn, then you will be asked to consume a specific amount of lactose. Most doctors use the traditional lactose-and-water solution, though some use ordinary milk for a more natural reaction.

One advantage of the blood glucose test is that it usually doesn't take as long as the breath hydrogen test; blood samples are drawn every half hour following the consumption of lactose, and most patients are finished within two hours or so. Another advantage is that testing labs don't need expensive equipment to measure glucose levels in blood samples, so just about any laboratory can do it.

Q: If the blood glucose test is so good, why don't doctors use it more often?

A: Because it's just not as accurate at identifying lactose intolerance as the breath hydrogen test. While the lactose-intolerance test can identify changes (or a lack of changes) in blood glucose levels following the consumption of lactose, this in itself is not necessarily an accurate indicator of lactose intolerance because such readings can be influenced by a wide range of factors, including differences in the time it takes the stomach to move lactose into the small intestines and individual blood glucose metabolism rates. It has other problems, too. Taking blood from veins or capillaries, for example, often results in incorrect readings. And it's ineffective on diabetics, who must struggle daily to balance their blood glucose levels properly.

Ultimately, the hydrogen breath test proved to be easier and less invasive than the blood glucose test—and far more accurate. The blood glucose test is still used as a diagnostic tool for other disorders, such as diabetes, but is seen less and less in the diagnosis of lactose intolerance. Today, it's used primarily in cases in which the hydrogen breath test isn't feasible, if there is a strong indication of non-hydrogen-producing bacteria, or if a doctor does not have ready access to a lab with the technology necessary for hydrogen analysis.

Q: I was diagnosed as lactose intolerant more than a decade ago via a blood glucose test, even though my symptoms don't always match those commonly associated with the condition. Is it possible that I was inaccurately diagnosed?

A: Yes, it's possible. In the past, most doctors relied on the glucose blood test because, despite its somewhat poor accuracy rate, it was the best they had at the time. Since you suspect that you may have been inaccurately diagnosed, ask your primary care doctor to conduct a breath hydrogen test as confirmation. In most cases, it should be able to tell you once and for all whether you truly are lactose intolerant.

Q: What other kinds of tests are used to diagnose lactose intolerance?

A: There are a number of them, few of which are in continued use for one reason or another. Some, such as tests that measure carbon dioxide levels in the breath, were found to be unreliable. Others, such as those requiring X-rays or radioactive tracers, posed too great a health risk to the patient.

One intriguing test that has found greater favor in Europe than in the United States looks for galactose, the other simple sugar created by the digestion of lactose. Measuring galactose levels as an indicator of lactose intolerance makes sense because unlike glucose, which can be derived from a number of different sources, galactose can be created only through the digestion of lactose.

Galactose can be difficult to measure because it travels quickly from the intestines to the liver, where it is converted into glucose. But researchers discovered a way to halt that conversion and keep galactose in the bloodstream or have it transfer into the urine. The result: A quick and easy test that offers a very reliable indicator of lactose intolerance within 30 to 40 minutes after lactose has been consumed.

The primary reason this test is not used more often in the United States is that it requires ethanol to get the liver to temporarily stop metabolizing galactose. Ethanol is the form of alcohol found in most alcoholic beverages, and the galactose test requires an amount equivalent to that found in a single beer (though smaller amounts are used in children). In Europe, where this test is commonly used, the alcoholic equivalent of one beer is thought of as inconsequential, and most clinical studies seem to agree with that evaluation. But here in the United States, alcohol—even when used medically—is frowned upon, and little information on this test can be found in the medical literature. Rather than risk controversy, most doctors avoid the galactose test in favor of the hydrogen breath test, even though European studies suggest that the galactose test is more accurate in diagnosing lactose intolerance.

Q: Instead of monitoring levels of blood glucose or breath hydrogen, why not go directly to the source and measure the amount of lactase produced by the intestines? That, it seems, would be the most accurate diagnosis of lactose intolerance.

A: You're right—a measurement of lactase levels would, indeed, be an accurate determination of lactose intolerance. Unfortunately, this is easier said than done.

There are no reliable tests to determine the extent of lactase production. It can't be measured by looking at blood or urine or any other easy-to-obtain bodily fluid. The only way to do it is to go directly to the source— the jejunum—and remove a section for analysis. There are two ways to approach this procedure, known as a biopsy. The first would be to surgically open the patient, find the jejunum, and lop off a piece. Since lactose intolerance is not a life-threatening disorder, most doctors consider this extreme and will not do it. The alternative is to maneuver a probe, either through the mouth down or from the rectum upward to the jejunum, and take a look that way. Again, this is easier said than done. Whichever course you take, getting to the jejunum is a difficult task that takes time and skill.

Once at the jejunum, the doctor may snip off a couple of small pieces of intestinal tissue and send them to a laboratory for testing and microscopic analysis. The laboratory pathologists won't actually see any lactase, but they can look for damage to the lining of the intestine, known as the mucosa, that could indicate poor lactase production and thus poor lactose digestion. If a person has gradually developed lactose intolerance over time, his intestinal tissue may appear completely healthy, yet he may still suffer from symptoms. In cases such as these, microscopic examination can be used to measure the extent of lactase activity, or to determine the ratio of lactase to sucrase, the enzyme that digests sucrose. The latter is the best measure, doctors say, because lactase activity can vary throughout the intestine but the ratio between the two enzymes remains pretty much constant.

An intestinal biopsy offers a very accurate diagnosis of lactose intolerance, but it is rarely done simply to confirm suspicion of the condition. Because of the invasiveness, risk, and inherent discomfort of the procedure, along with the fact that a breath hydrogen test is almost as accurate, intestinal biopsies are usually reserved for more serious concerns, such as intestinal polyps or cancer.

Q: Is the breath hydrogen test also effective in diagnosing lactose intolerance in babies and children?

A: Absolutely. The hydrogen breath test has been shown effective in children as young as six months (the age at which many children start to develop intestine-damaging viral infections), and is the treatment of choice because it is so easy, painless, and noninvasive. The only difference between performing the test on children and adults is the amount of lactose that must be ingested; obviously, children and infants are given much smaller amounts. Unlike adults, children must fast for about six hours before the test, but that's generally not a problem. If a child is old enough, he can blow through the mouthpiece and fill balloons just like an adult. In children too young to perform such a task, a nasal prong or infant face mask may be required.

One of the few times a hydrogen breath test may be ineffective in babies or children is if extended bouts of diarrhea have greatly reduced the population of the bacteria in the colon that produce the gas. In such cases, the test is usually postponed until the diarrhea has eased for several days and colonic bacteria have had a chance to multiply. This is typically signaled by the recurrence of lactose-intolerance symptoms.

Q: How is lactose intolerance determined in babies too young or otherwise unable to take a breath hydrogen test?

A: If a doctor suspects that a child's digestive symptoms are being caused by something very serious, she may recommend an intestinal biopsy. However, this is quite rare and suggested only in extreme cases. In situations in which it appears that lactose intolerance is the culprit and a breath hydrogen test is inappropriate, the doctor may perform a stool acidity test. This is a simple test that can be done at bedside using an ordinary piece of litmus paper or other instrument; it doesn't require that samples be sent away to a laboratory for analysis.

A stool acidity test is a good indicator of lactose intolerance in children because only carbohydrates create acidic stools, and the only carbohydrate in mother's milk and most commercial formulas is lactose. As we've learned, undigested lactose is fermented by bacteria in the colon, creating lactic acid and other short-chain fatty acids that can be easily detected in a stool sample. In addition, glucose may be present in the sample as a result of unabsorbed lactose in the colon. But while helpful in indicating a potential lactose problem, a stool acidity test is not accurate enough to be used as a general test for lactose intolerance. Most doctors use a stool acidity test only as a guide in determining whether to place a child on a reduced-lactose or lactose-free diet.

Another alternative in determining lactose intolerance in babies and children is measuring stool sugar levels via chemical analysis or the use of special tablets. But like the stool acidity test, this technique is not extremely reliable and is generally used only to corroborate a suspected diagnosis of poor lactose digestion.

Q: I've been out of work for a while and thus I have to watch my finances. I think I may have lactose intolerance, but at the moment I don't have the money to see a doctor. Can I do a home test for self-diagnosis?
A: Yes. If your symptoms are fairly indicative of lactose intolerance, you can save yourself some money, time, and inconvenience by diagnosing yourself at home. But keep in mind that a self-test is not as reliable or as accurate as a breath hydrogen test, and that a self-test should be done only if there are absolutely no symptoms of more serious intestinal problems, such as cancer. (See Chapter Two for a detailed discussion of colon cancer.)

There are two tests you can do yourself: the lactose challenge and the lactose-free test. The lactose challenge involves drinking approximately a quart of milk in one fifteen-minute sitting, then monitoring your symptoms. A quart of milk provides almost the same amount of lactose as the solution used in clinical testing (approximately 50 grams), so it should easily trigger noticeable symptoms—usually within two hours—if you really are lactose intolerant. Make sure you perform this test on a day when you have no other plans, just in case symptoms strike more severely than anticipated and you find yourself racing for the bathroom.

The lactose-free test is just the opposite of the lactose challenge. Rather than forcing your system to deal with a sudden, heavy dose of lactose, the lactose-free diet eliminates as much lactose as possible on the theory that if you are lactose intolerant, your symptoms will slow or disappear.

For best results, doctors suggest adhering to a lactose-free diet for a minimum of five days. This should be a sufficient length of time for a noticeable decrease in symptoms if lactose intolerance is, indeed, your problem. Of course, it's important that you maintain a strong vigil. Many common foods contain hidden lactose (see Chapter Seven for a comprehensive discussion of this issue) and it's easy to consume lactose without realizing it. During your "lactose fast," stick with fresh fruits and vegetables, fish, poultry, and lean meat. You should also avoid eating out during this period. If you must use a processed food, read the ingredients closely to make sure it does not contain milk products, including whey. It can also be helpful to choose foods with a kosher label. According to Jewish dietary laws, items identified as "pareve" or "parve" must contain no dairy or meat. Kosher meat items, such as kosher chicken noodle soup, will also contain no dairy because milk and meat cannot be combined. Eating Asian cuisine can be equally beneficial, because most Asian dishes contain very little, if any, dairy products.

As the days go by, monitor your symptoms and note

any obvious changes, including occurrence and severity. If you really are lactose intolerant, you should notice a dramatic reduction in symptoms from one day to the next. After the test period, gradually reintroduce lactose-containing products back into your diet. But don't over-do it—too much lactose at once could result in a major flare-up. By slowly introducing milk products, you can determine just how much of your favorite lactose-containing foods you can eat before symptoms occur. Most lactose-intolerant people find that they can eat almost anything they want as long as they don't go over a certain amount.

Let me reiterate: Self-testing is a good way to screen for lactose intolerance, but it's not as accurate or as definitive as clinical testing. If, after conducting the tests discussed above, you're still not certain, see your doctor.

"I had long suspected that I was lactose intolerant, and I pretty much confirmed that when I took the lactose-free test for a week," notes Peter, a 33-year-old firefighter. "I kept a food diary for a while and found that I experienced mild to moderate intestinal problems, primarily gas and bloating, after I ate certain kinds of foods. Just to be sure, I eliminated as much lactose from my diet as I could and noticed an almost immediate improvement. No painful gas, no bloating, no diarrhea. As far as I was concerned, my self-diagnosis was correct, and I saw no need to go to a doctor for a breath hydrogen test.

"After five days off lactose, I very gradually started adding small amounts of dairy products to my diet. Some foods caused more problems than others, but I found that I could eat just about anything as long as I didn't pig out on it. That's how I keep my lactose intolerance under control."

Q: I've spent years under the assumption that my digestive distress was the result of a milk allergy. Now I'm not so sure. What are the real symptoms of a milk allergy and how is the condition typically diagnosed?

A: A true allergy to cow's milk (or, more specifically, to certain proteins found in cow's milk) is a relatively rare health condition—and one that is completely different from lactose intolerance. As noted earlier in this book, an allergy to cow's milk protein (CMP) is an immunologic response, whereas lactose intolerance is the result of the body's inability to digest lactose properly. Both are dairy-related, but that's where the similarity stops.

In a healthy individual, food proteins are broken down during digestion into their component amino acids, which the body absorbs and uses for maintenance. But if whole proteins accidentally find their way into the bloodstream, the body perceives them as unwanted invaders (like germs) and starts manufacturing large numbers of antibodies to fight them. These antibodies are present in the bloodstream, and produce an allergic reaction whenever those specific proteins are found. It doesn't take a lot to get the body going, allergy experts note. Even very small amounts of cow's milk protein can result in severe allergy symptoms.

There are many symptoms of a true milk allergy. Symptoms usually include protracted diarrhea, vomiting, and bloody diarrhea caused by local damage of the small and large bowel. Occasionally, symptoms of milk allergy may be systemic (affecting the body as a whole). Skin reactions to milk allergy can include an itchy, red rash; eczema; hives; and swelling of the lips, mouth, tongue, and face. In extreme cases, the throat may swell up and block the individual's airway (a phenomenon known medically as anaphylactic shock) if emergency medical attention isn't received promptly. So milk and other food allergies aren't just bothersome; they can even be life-threatening.

Stomach and intestinal reactions to a milk allergy often mimic those of lactose intolerance, which is why a lot of people with milk allergies think they're just lactose intolerant, and vice versa. Common intestinal symptoms include vomiting, gas, cramping, and diarrhea. In addition, milk-allergy sufferers may also experience watery or itchy eyes, runny nose, sneezing, coughing, shortness of breath, and even depression, anxiety, fatigue, migraine headaches, and insomnia.

One of the biggest differences between a milk allergy and lactose intolerance is the rate at which symptoms occur. Milk-allergy symptoms usually appear within minutes of consuming cow's milk, while symptoms of lactose intolerance may not present themselves for several hours.

CMP allergy can be easily diagnosed by a doctor using the standard allergy testing technique of gently scratching the skin and applying a small amount of the suspected allergen (in this case, milk) to the scratch. If a person is truly allergic, a raised welt will appear at the scratch site within 15 minutes or so. Mothers can verify a suspected milk allergy in young children by placing a drop of milk on the youngsters' skin (there's no need to make a scratch) and watching for the development of a hive or welt. If this occurs, see your pediatrician for a confirming clinical allergy test, as well as information on allergy management.

In the majority of cases, a milk allergy can be successfully managed by carefully avoiding products containing cow's milk protein, such as whole milk, ice cream, butter, and most cheeses. Sometimes CMP allergy is permanent, but most cases—especially those that manifest in early childhood—gradually disappear as the individual ages.

If the symptoms of a milk allergy—or any food allergy—are extremely severe and result in anaphylactic shock (swelling of the throat resulting in a blocked airway), it's a good idea to keep an allergy-response kit in your house. Such kits are available through your doctor or at larger drug stores and contain a fast-acting dose of epinephrine, which quickly reverses the effects of anaphylactic shock. Individuals who are very allergic to bees often keep such kits with them in case of emergency. If an allergy-response kit is unavailable and someone goes into anaphylaxis as a result of a food allergy, an over-the-counter antihistamine such as Benadryl can help reduce the effects of the reaction until the person can be taken to the hospital.

There is also a condition known as cow milk protein intolerance, which is somewhat different from lactose intolerance. CMP intolerance is often seen in young children, and symptoms, which usually affect just the gastrointestinal tract, typically take longer to present than those resulting from a CMP allergy. In the majority of cases, CMP intolerance disappears as a child ages and her digestive tract grows stronger and more resilient.

Q: My sister recently gave birth to a gorgeous baby girl. The delivering obstetrician told my sister that the baby has something called glucose-galactose malabsorption. Is that just another name for lactose intolerance?

A: No, it's a completely different condition. Glucose-galactose malabsorption results when lactose is adequately broken down by lactase, but the resulting simple sugars—glucose and galactose—cannot be absorbed by the body. It's an extremely rare condition, but it can pose serious health problems, especially among newborns such as your niece. Luckily, doctors are able to diagnose it at birth and place infants with the condition on more easily absorbed fructose-based formulas. Most of the symptoms of glucose-galactose malabsorption, including chronic diarrhea, usually disappear by age 5 as the body learns to adapt to the condition.

Though seen primarily in newborns, glucose-galactose malabsorption occasionally occurs in older children and adults. In such cases, diet must be carefully monitored to make sure it does not contain any lactose. Other carbohydrates may also have to be excluded.

A close cousin of glucose-galactose malabsorption is another rare condition known as galactosemia. As in glucose-galactose malabsorption, lactose is properly broken down by lactase, but the special liver enzyme that converts galactose into glucose is missing or insufficient. Again, this is most commonly seen in newborns and is genetic in origin. Symptoms include persistent vomiting, weight loss, jaundice, and liver problems, and usually present themselves a few days after a newborn has been on mother's milk or any lactose-rich commercial formula.

If left untreated, the unconverted galactose will build up in the blood and various body tissues, resulting in a number of health problems that can include liver damage and even mental retardation.

Because of the seriousness of galactosemia, doctors usually diagnose it at birth by doing a quick screen of blood taken from the umbilical cord. If galactosemia is detected, the infant must be placed on a lactose-free formula, and must avoid all lactose-containing foods for the rest of its life. Even a small amount of lactose could prove dangerous.

detected the small amount of lactose on a food-by-food
basis, and most every product containing lactose for the
rest of his life. Even a small amount of lactose could
prove dangerous.

FOUR

How is Lactose
Intolerance Treated?

WHEN A BREATH HYDROGEN TEST REVEALED THAT
Yvette was lactose intolerant, the 42-year-old freelance
musician broke down and cried.

"I'm a dairy nut, and all I could think of when my
doctor broke the news was that I would no longer be
able to enjoy any of my favorite foods," Yvette recalls.
"I love milk. I love cheese. And I practically live for
ice cream. It's my favorite comfort food. For years, I've
had a large bowl every evening before I go to bed. I
didn't want lactose intolerance to prevent me from consuming dairy. It seemed very unfair."

Yvette was able to enjoy lactose-containing foods
without a problem until about two years ago. Suddenly
she noticed that she became gassy and bloated if she ate
too much ice cream. Over time, the gas and bloating
were accompanied by frequent bouts of explosive diarrhea. Cutting back on the amount of dairy products she

consumed helped a little, but soon Yvette was afraid to eat any at all.

"I was certain almost from the beginning that I had developed lactose intolerance, though I really didn't want to admit it to myself," Yvette says. "I read about the condition in a number of magazines, and my symptoms were practically a textbook example. Still, deep in my heart, I was hopeful that my problem might be something else; something that would be easy to fix and allow me to continue eating dairy products as I had in the past."

Yvette finally saw her primary care doctor at the urging of her boyfriend, who was concerned about the increasing frequency of Yvette's digestive distress. The doctor took her medical history, gave her a complete physical, then discussed Yvette's symptoms at length to determine if she could be suffering from something more serious than an inability to digest dairy products. Concluding that Yvette was in otherwise good health, the doctor recommended a breath hydrogen test to confirm his diagnosis of lactose intolerance. It came back positive.

"The test didn't bother me, but the diagnosis did," Yvette notes. "I told my doctor about my concerns and how much I loved dairy foods, and he quickly reassured me that the condition was usually easy to control and that I wouldn't have to give up all dairy products. He told me most people with lactose intolerance can still enjoy their favorite lactose-containing foods in moderation, or with the assistance of lactase enzyme tablets."

Following the breath hydrogen test, Yvette placed herself on a lactose-free diet for a week. She avoided all foods containing lactose, and read product labels very carefully to ensure that she didn't ingest any hidden lactose. Not surprisingly, her symptoms decreased dramatically, and all but disappeared by the end of the week.

"Then, with my doctor's encouragement, I slowly added lactose-containing foods to my diet. I kept the portions small, and was delighted when I didn't show any symptoms after a small bowl of my favorite ice cream. A few days later, however, I ate my usual portion and immediately realized I had pushed things too far. I also had trouble with whole milk and a few other products."

Yvette determined through trial and error just how much of her favorite foods she could eat without inducing symptoms and is careful never to exceed that amount. She also occasionally relies on commercial lactase tablets to make digestion a little easier, especially if she is dining out or at a party where lactose could be hidden in just about anything.

"I quickly realized that my fears regarding lactose intolerance were unjustified," Yvette says now. "My understanding of lactose intolerance wasn't completely correct, and I made a lot of erroneous assumptions. Like most people with the condition, I can eat almost anything I want as long as I use a little common sense. I can't binge on milk and ice cream, but I can still enjoy them in moderation. And believe me, that's better than nothing!"

Yvette is just one of many people with lactose intolerance who have found the condition relatively easy to manage as long as they don't overdo their favorite lactose-containing foods. In this chapter, we'll discuss the various ways lactose intolerance can be treated, including the use of various lactase enzyme items and lactose-reduced food products.

Q: I come from a long line of lactose-intolerant individuals, and after two years of occasional symptoms have finally reached the point where I need
to do something about my condition. My question
is: How effective is dietary control in the management of lactose intolerance? Could simply monitoring my diet be all I need to avoid symptoms?

A: It depends on the extent of your condition. If you are
severely lactose intolerant, you may need more help than
mere dietary control can offer. However, a sizable percentage of people with mild to moderate lactose intolerance find that they can effectively manage their
condition through dietary control alone, and don't need
to rely on lactase enzymes or other aides.

For most individuals with lactose intolerance, dietary
control is a simple matter of trial and error—eating increasing amounts of lactose until symptoms appear, then
backing off a little. Start by going on a lactose-free diet
(or as close as you can come) for a week or more. Avoid
all known dairy products and read the ingredients of
processed foods to make sure you aren't ingesting hidden lactose. Within days, you should notice a dramatic
reduction in symptoms at mealtime. They may even go
away completely.

Once your system is sufficiently cleansed, gradually
reintroduce lactose-containing foods to your diet. Start
with small amounts—perhaps a single scoop of ice
cream rather than a heaping bowl—and monitor your
symptoms. If none occur, increase the amount in small,
measurable increments over a period of days until you
notice the onset of symptoms. That is your breakthrough
point, the amount of lactose that your intestines can no
longer comfortably digest. By decreasing that amount,
you'll know exactly how much of a given product you

can enjoy without having to worry about intestinal distress.

Dietary control of lactose intolerance can be time-consuming, but most people with the condition find it worthwhile because it enables them to continue eating their favorite dairy products, though usually in smaller amounts. It's also more cost-effective because they don't have to buy commercial enzyme products designed to make the digestion of lactose easier.

Culinary boredom can be reduced by incorporating nondairy alternatives into your menu. Soy products, for example, can often be substituted for cow's milk in many recipes, and a wide variety of nondairy alternatives are available for people with lactose intolerance, such as Tofutti (an ice-cream-like product made of tofu) instead of ice cream. Certain low-lactose international cuisines can also make dinner time more fun and enjoyable. Chinese, Japanese, and Thai food make a tasty change of pace, and are acceptable for people with lactose intolerance because most Asian dishes use little, if any, cow's milk.

Q: Is there a downside to dietary control as a management tool for lactose intolerance?
A: It's definitely not for everyone. Individuals who are severely lactose intolerant, or who experience incapacitating symptoms after ingesting even small amounts of lactose, may have no choice but to avoid almost all dairy products, or add lactase enzyme tablets or liquid to the lactose-containing foods they do eat. This shouldn't be considered a personal failing. Everyone is different, and we often require varying degrees of treatment for certain health problems. Ten people with nearsightedness, for example, may need ten different degrees of correction

based on the individual severity of their vision problem. The strengths of their glasses are different, yet they are all nearsighted. Lactose intolerance is the same way. Some people are only mildly affected, while others are affected very severely.

In addition, some people with lactose intolerance try their hand at dietary control, but eventually give it up in favor of lactase supplements because they find dietary control too confining. They may not like being limited in the amount of lactose-containing foods they can eat, or they may find the constant monitoring of ingredients too time-consuming. And that's fine. Dietary control works for a lot of people with lactose intolerance, but it's not the only answer.

If you're unsure whether dietary control for lactose intolerance is for you, talk with your primary care doctor or gastroenterologist. Your doctor can explain in simple terms what would be involved in your particular case, and whether or not it's something you should consider.

Q: I'm pretty severely lactose intolerant. Even small amounts of certain dairy products mess me up for hours. I tried dietary control, but found it just too difficult to maintain so my doctor has suggested I start using lactase supplements. I'm not really familiar with these products. Could you give us a little bit of history?

A: It used to be that if you were lactose intolerant, you simply avoided milk and other dairy products, usually at the expense of some of your favorite foods. But no more. Thanks to lactase enzyme supplements, most people with lactose intolerance can continue to enjoy lactose-containing foods with a minimum of symptoms, or no symptoms at all.

Perfecting lactase supplementation as we know it today was no easy task. One answer briefly considered was the manufacture of artificial lactase, a synthetic form of the naturally occurring enzyme. However, the logistics of such an endeavor almost immediately proved too formidable for even the most high-tech pharmaceutical company. Had it been accomplished, the resulting products would no doubt have been too costly for most people with lactose intolerance to afford.

Thankfully, nature provided us with a less expensive alternative. As we know, lactase production is not just a function of intestinal tissue—a wide number of microorganisms also produce lactase as part of their ability to ferment lactose. Some of these microorganisms are found in the intestines, but there are many others. Researchers at the Dutch pharmaceutical company Gist-Brocades realized that such organisms could be easily cultivated and the lactase they produced harvested in quantities large enough to make it affordable to everyone.

But which microorganism was best for the job? Scientists at Gist-Brocades evaluated a lot of them and finally decided on a unique dairy yeast known as *Kluyveromyces lactis*, which was commonly used in Russia for the manufacture of various fermented milk products. This organism produced lactase in large amounts, and the resulting enzyme proved quite effective in easing symptoms among those with lactose intolerance.

The first commercial product, called Maxilact, was released in the early 1970s. It was a powder added to fresh milk to break down lactose into its component sugars, glucose and galactose, for easy digestion. A liquid form was developed in 1979 but, like the powder, it was used primarily to create reduced-lactose milk and other dairy products. An enzyme pill that people with lactose intolerance could take along with dairy products wouldn't be developed for a while. Still, reduced-lactose dairy products were definitely a step in the right direction, and a blessing to people who until that time had been forced to give up dairy products altogether.

If there's an American savior for the lactose intolerant, it's Alan Klingerman, the heir to a New Jersey dairy company and, perhaps more importantly, a dairy science major at Cornell University. Klingerman realized the various health problems associated with dairy products and tried to find effective answers. One of his first products was a sugar-reduced ice cream for people with diabetes. Lactose intolerance was another concern for Klingerman who, in 1974, bought exclusive American marketing rights to Maxilact under the brand name Lact-Aid.

Klingerman first sold the powdered enzyme through mail order, then through health food stores and pharmacies across the United States. When the liquid form of the enzyme became available, Klingerman produced special "Lact-Aid" lactose-reduced milk and other dairy products and sold them through a small number of supermarkets. These items were fairly successful, but the enzyme powder and drops literally flew off the shelves as people with lactose intolerance discovered that they could once again enjoy milk and other dairy products merely by adding Lact-Aid to them.

In 1985, the dream of lactose-intolerance sufferers everywhere came true when Klingerman added Lact-Aid pills to his burgeoning line of products. Finally, people with the aggravating digestive condition could eat almost anything they wanted merely by popping an enzyme pill.

Life suddenly became a lot easier for the lactose intolerant, and Alan Klingerman became a wealthy man.

Lact-Aid—now known commercially as Lactaid— wasn't the only product on the market for people with lactose intolerance, but it was by far the most popular. In 1990, however, Lactaid received its first real competition when Dairy Ease hit the market. With strong financial backing, the company promoted its products to dairy-wary consumers with money-saving coupons, magazine advertising, and national television commercials. Lactaid found itself forced to fight back to retain its market share, and the battle was on. The resulting advertising/educational blitz brought lactose intolerance to the forefront of the American consciousness, and made more people aware of the condition than ever before. It also resulted in millions of dollars in sales of lactase-based and lactose-reduced products. A handful of smaller companies took advantage of the burgeoning market, but Lactaid and Dairy Ease remain the biggest manufacturers of products for the management of lactose intolerance.

Q: Why did it take so long for a lactase pill to reach the market?
A: Because adding lactase to milk to break down lactose is not nearly as complicated as finding the right kind of lactase for the human digestive system—or finding a way to deliver it safely to the intestines.

It must be remembered that while all lactase breaks down lactose, the many forms of lactase produced by microorganisms have wildly divergent properties. For example, no two forms of lactase are effective in the same conditions of acidity or temperature, so researchers had to find the one that appeared to be most effective within the strict parameters of the human digestive system. (Human lactase is designed to be most efficient in the intestines, which have a near-constant temperature of 98.6°F and a relatively neutral acidity rating of 7 due to the alkaline compounds produced by the liver and pancreas specifically to neutralize corrosive stomach acid.)

The lactase produced by *Kluyveromyces lactis* comes very close to fitting the bill, showing effectiveness in both the acidity and temperature of the human intestines. However, it just didn't work well in pill form because stomach acids caused the enzyme to break down before it could reach the lower digestive tract, where it was needed.

The search for the most efficient form of lactase led researchers to a fungus known as *Aspergillis niger*, which manufactures lactase that is able to tolerate the acidic environment of the stomach. However, it also prefers temperatures around the 140°F mark, which is considerably higher than the human body's core temperature of 98.6°F. As a result, this form of lactase tends to lose a considerable amount of activity at body temperature, though it still has a lot of commercial potential and is sometimes used in the manufacture of lactase pills.

Hoping they could find a form of lactase even better suited for use in the human digestive tract, scientists finally turned to a fungus known as *Aspergillis oryzae*, which is a close cousin to *Aspergillis niger*. When taken with food, the lactase produced by this specific microorganism proved quite successful at both surviving the harsh conditions of the stomach and breaking down lactose in human small intestines. Not surprisingly, it is the lactase of choice for most commercial oral lactase supplements.

Q: Are commercial lactase pills considered drugs or nutritional supplements?

A: The U.S. Food and Drug Administration (FDA) currently classifies lactase as a food supplement, which means lactase products do not have to meet the same stringent standards as drugs. However, there has been some talk about reclassification. Advocates of such a move say that relabeling enzymes as drugs would result in a more uniform measure of lactase activity and thus allow comparisons between various products. As it now stands, there is little uniformity within the industry, and consumers are often confused and frustrated by such issues as pill strength and expiration time.

Right now, nearly all commercial lactase supplements list their strengths in one of two distinct units—FCC units (FCC stands for Food Chemicals Codex, and is also known as a Neutral Lactase Unit) and the more commonly recognized milligrams (typically abbreviated as "mg"). Almost immediately, problems arise when it comes to evaluating competing products because FCC units and milligrams cannot be compared or converted. Comparing two products that list their strengths in milligrams can be just as difficult because lactase is sold in both pharmaceutical grade and food grade. Food-grade lactase is generally less expensive because it contains harmless fillers that dilute the activity of lactase per unit of weight. In other words, you often need more of a food-grade lactase supplement to get the job done because it doesn't contain as much active ingredient as a product made with pharmaceutical-grade lactase.

Indeed, the strength and effectiveness of various supplements can vary widely, as noted in a 1994 study of lactase products from around the world, reported in the *Scandinavian Journal of Gastroenterology*. Noted the researchers: "To hydrolyze about 90 percent of the lactose contained in one liter of milk, the following amounts of enzymes are needed: 0.25 g of Maxilact LX 5000 produced by Gist-Brocades NV; or 2 ml of Lactozyme 3000 L, produced by Novo Industries of Denmark; or 2.6 g of Lactaid (liquid form), produced by SugarLo Co., Inc.; or 0.64 g Lactase A (Takamine) by Miles Lab, Elkhart, Indiana; or 0.4 g of Lactase N produced by GB Fermentation Products Co., USA."

Q: I find all of this scientific language pretty confusing. Is it safe to assume that all commercial lactase products are essentially the same and equally effective?
A: No.There can be substantial differences in effectiveness between two seemingly similar products. Predicating factors can include the quality of the lactase in the product (whether it is food grade or pharmaceutical grade), the amount of lactase in each pill or capsule, and how long the bottles have been on the store shelf.

Lactase products work—that much we do know. But finding the right product or amount for your particular condition may require some trial and error. Your doctor may be able to make some recommendations. You may also find it helpful to talk to other people with lactose intolerance who take lactase supplements with their food. Their experiences may be able to save you considerable time and effort.

Q: What are the advantages of lactase pills over other products for the control of lactose intolerance?
A: Convenience is the biggest advantage, say the people who use commercial lactase supplements. They are rel-

atively inexpensive, easy to use, and they travel anywhere, so you can use them while dining out. Best of all, enzyme supplements make the digestion of almost any lactose-containing food easier. Milk is the most obvious, but lactase supplements work with just about anything, which means you don't have to monitor your diet quite as closely. For those who truly enjoy dairy foods, or anything containing lactose, enzyme pills can be a real lifesaver.

The word *pill*, however, is a bit of misnomer. Lactase supplements come in a variety of forms, including capsules (standard, softgel, and openable), caplets and chewable tablets (not to mention powder that can be added to milk and other dairy products). The product that works best for you depends on your personal needs and habits. Some people have no trouble taking a hard pill, while others find caplets or chewable tablets easier. And many prefer openable capsules because they like being able to sprinkle the enzyme on their food (don't worry—it usually doesn't affect the taste). Again, it may require some trial and error before you find the one product that is best suited for you.

Q: What is the most effective way to take a lactase supplement? I want to make sure it works.
A: It's always wise to read the directions before taking any new dietary supplement. But in general, lactase should be consumed with your meals. Many people with lactose intolerance take their supplements a few minutes before sitting down to eat. Others wait until they take the first bite of food. And some don't take their lactase until they start eating something they know contains lactose. There's really no absolute "right" way to take lactase supplements, though most doctors suggest taking a

lactase pill immediately before taking your first bite because food will help buffer the enzyme in the pill as it passes through the stomach. Taking a pill or capsule a few minutes before dining is usually okay (make sure you check the directions) but you don't want to wait too long because the undiluted juices in the stomach may diminish the effectiveness of the enzyme before it has a chance to make its way to the small intestines.

Q: How many lactase pills should I take with my meals? I don't want to take too few—or too many.
A: That's a good question, and one that's difficult to answer. The number of pills, capsules, or tablets required for the control of lactose intolerance depends on a number of factors, including your degree of lactose intolerance, the amount and purity of the lactase in each pill, the age of the pills (pills that have been lying around for a while usually aren't as effective as newer ones), the types of lactose-containing foods you're eating, the amount of lactose in those foods (some are more lactose-rich than others), whether lactose-containing foods are consumed with other foods, and the length of time over which they are eaten. Other considerations include the speed at which food moves out of your stomach and into the intestines, the general condition of your intestines (those in poor condition may require more pills), and how quickly food moves through your intestines.

Most products offer a general dosage guide, but (here's that phrase again) a little trial and error may be required before you discover the best dose for you when eating a particular food. Popping pills throughout a high-lactose meal, such as a double cheese pizza, is probably a good idea, but after a while, you may become a victim of the law of diminishing return. Three pills may work better than two, but you won't necessarily increase effectiveness by taking five or six. After a while, it's all a moot point.

When taken properly, lactase supplements are almost always very effective in aiding the digestion of lactose and eliminating the telltale symptoms of lactose intolerance. Study after study has shown this, and word of mouth among those with lactose intolerance is equally strong. Without adding too much hype, it's accurate to say that lactase pills can make life fun again for the majority of individuals with lactose intolerance.

Q: Is it possible to take too much lactase? Can you overdose on these supplements?
A: You can take more lactase than you need to do the job, but there's no evidence that you can overdose on the enzyme. When lactase pills first hit the market, the accompanying literature warned users against taking more than a certain amount because investigators hadn't done much research in that area and were unsure of the potential consequences of ingesting large quantities of the enzyme. But over the years, researchers have become more and more certain of the safety of such products. In fact, laboratory animals have been fed large amounts of lactase—sometimes in doses up to 50 percent of their food supply—and experienced no problems at all.

This shouldn't come as a surprise. After all, lactase is naturally produced by the human body and serves a very valuable function. There is no evidence that the body can produce too much lactase, or that such an amount could even be defined. More importantly, the lactase in commercial enzyme supplements does not go anywhere but the digestive tract, where it is eventually broken down into easily (and safely) absorbed protein fragments.

But while lactase itself is perfectly safe, there could be a very minor safety concern regarding the fillers contained in many lactase products made with food-grade enzyme. According to allergy specialists, a small number of individuals could be allergic or overly sensitive to these compounds, resulting in allergy symptoms. There have also been a very small number of reports in the medical literature regarding an allergic reaction to the fungus used to manufacture lactase enzyme. In one report, noted in the *Journal of Allergy and Clinical Immunology*, a man experienced burning and swelling of his throat with difficulty swallowing after taking a commercial lactase capsule.

If you experience any allergy symptoms that could be related to your lactase supplements, stop taking them immediately and consult with your doctor for safer alternatives. Again, this is a minor issue that affects a very small percentage of people, but it still deserves a mention.

Finally, please don't consider this an endorsement for rampant lactase consumption! Just because there is no clinical evidence that high doses of the enzyme are harmful doesn't mean you should start popping lactase pills as if they were candy. Read the directions on the packaging and do your own trials until you find out the right dose for you—then stick with it. There's no need to take more than what works.

Q: I've just started taking lactase supplements with meals to control the symptoms of lactose intolerance, and sometimes I forget about the pills until

it's too late. Is it okay to take lactase after I've eaten a lactose-rich meal? Could it still help me?
A: Let's just say it couldn't hurt. Most lactase supplements are designed to be taken during a meal, but some studies have found that taking lactase shortly after the fact can occasionally help minimize lactose intolerance symptoms, if not prevent them completely.

If you forget to take your lactase pills during a meal, try to take them immediately after. You may still experience some gas and bloating, but it probably won't be as severe as if you didn't take the supplements. Bottom line: You have little to lose and a lot to gain.

Many people with lactose intolerance find it helpful to keep lactase pills with them at all times, just to be safe. A variety of high-tech pill containers are available to help you remember to take your pills, including some that sound an alarm at specified mealtimes. It also helps to have family members remind you when it appears that you have forgotten. The more people involved, the greater the chance you'll take your lactase when you need it the most.

Q: Can I count on lactase supplements to provide the same level of relief at every meal, no matter what I eat?
A: Lactase is effective in preventing the symptoms of lactose intolerance by enabling the easy digestion of lactose, but it's not infallible. As noted earlier, a wide variety of factors all play a role in determining the effectiveness of the lactase you take with meals, including the severity of your condition, when you take the enzyme supplements, how much you take, the amount of active lactase in each dose, and the amount of lactose in the foods you're eating. It may take a while before you are able to gauge accurately how much lactase

you'll need at a given meal, but pretty soon you'll find yourself making the calculations with ease.

As a rule of thumb, the more lactose intolerant you are and the greater the amount of lactose in a particular meal, the more lactase you should consume with that meal—within reason. You don't want to go overboard because after a while the amount of lactase in your system will have reached maximum effectiveness.

If you've had good success with a particular lactase product, but suddenly realize it's not working as well as it used to, check the expiration date on the packaging. Some lactase products become unstable over time and gradually lose their effectiveness. If the product you're using is old and past its expiration date, throw it away and get a fresh package.

And, of course, if you suddenly develop more symptoms or your symptoms worsen noticeably despite your use of lactase supplements, see your doctor immediately. Your digestive condition could be something much worse than lactose intolerance. (See Chapter Five for a more thorough discussion of conditions that may mimic lactose intolerance.)

Q: I was recently diagnosed with lactose intolerance via a breath hydrogen test, and I thought it would be a good idea to experiment with various brands of lactase products to find the one best for me. However, a friend of mine who also has lactose intolerance told me my plan was a waste of time because all lactase products are essentially the same when it comes to effectiveness. Is this true?

A: No. Your friend is wrong. Studies have shown the potential for a wide range of effectiveness among commercial lactase products, so it's wise for you to experiment until you find the product and dose that works best for your specific condition. Remember: Everyone is different, and we all react to medication (including lactase supplements) in different ways.

One intriguing randomized, placebo-controlled experiment, reported in the *American Journal of Gastroenterology*, compared the effectiveness of three different products plus a placebo (an inactive sugar pill) in reducing symptoms among 10 diverse lactose intolerance sufferers following consumption of 1 cup of vanilla ice cream (approximately 18 grams of lactose). The products used in the study included three chewable Dairy Ease tablets, three Lactaid caplets, and two Lactrase capsules.

It might be assumed that all three products worked equally well, and that the placebo did nothing. However, the results of the study were decidedly mixed. The Lactaid caplets were the only supplements to significantly reduce breath hydrogen production, while Lactrase capsules reduced the maximum severity of pain and bloating, and the Dairy Ease chewable tablets reduced the maximum severity of pain. (The Lactaid caplets also reduced severity of symptoms, but not significantly). In addition, all three products dramatically reduced diarrhea, but none of them affected gas to a significant degree.

Despite the disparity in the clinical evaluation of symptom control, all of the products—including the placebo—made the test subjects feel better after eating lactose, the researchers noted, adding, ''Every lactase formulation was able to influence the symptomatic scores positively for each of the four individually assessed symptoms.''

There are a lot of possible explanations for the findings of this study, but the most obvious conclusion that can be drawn from it and similar studies is that no specific lactase product (or form) is perfect for everyone, and the smart consumer does some research and experimentation before settling on one brand over another. In addition to your own trial and error, it couldn't hurt to talk with your doctor to see what he recommends and why, as well as other individuals with lactose intolerance who also take lactase supplements. If you find that one particular product is mentioned considerably more often than others, it couldn't hurt to check it out.

Q: I've been experiencing symptoms of lactose intolerance for several months, and decided to take lactase pills with dinner last night to see if they would help. They didn't. My symptoms were just as bad as if I had taken nothing at all. What did I do wrong?

A: Probably nothing. The lactase you tried with your dinner may have proved ineffective for a number of reasons. The pills may have lost their efficacy because of their age, for example, or you tried a brand that simply wasn't compatible with your system. Most likely, though, you probably just didn't take enough. This is a very common problem among first-time lactase users—they take only one or two pills under the assumption that that's all they need, when in fact they actually need four or five for proper lactose digestion. This is especially true if you are eating a meal that's very high in lactose.

Give the pills another chance, but be aware that the brand you chose may not be the best for you. If you're using an off brand, consider switching to a better-known brand-name product. True, they cost a bit more, but it's worth it if they work well.

Another consideration is that you don't really have lactose intolerance. The fact that the pills you took had no effect at all on you suggests that you may have another type of digestive disorder. If you haven't had your condition confirmed by a breath hydrogen test or other exam, it's probably a good idea to do so. If the test is negative, your doctor can then suggest other tests to determine once and for all what your problem is and how it should be treated.

Q: I really enjoy milk and need the calcium to help ward off bone-weakening osteoporosis. However, I'm also lactose intolerant, which makes drinking milk in sufficient quantities rather difficult. I've searched without success for a commercial brand of low-lactose milk, so my doctor suggested I make my own by adding lactase drops to my regular brand. Could you tell me what this entails, and whether it really works? I don't want to spend a lot of money on a product only to find that I can't use it.

A: Lactase drops for making low-lactose milk at home is one of the oldest products available to people with lactose intolerance. Lactase powder was available before that, but the liquid drops quickly made the powder obsolete because the drops are more stable and much more convenient.

There are a variety of enzyme drops available on the commercial market, and they all work fairly well when it comes to reducing lactose levels in milk. Most contain lactase enzyme harvested from the yeast *K. lactis* in a harmless base and, when added to fresh milk, effectively break down lactose into its component sugars, glucose and galactose. Just five drops or so of most products will remove up to 70 percent of lactose in a quart of milk, but it doesn't happen immediately. The milk must sit in the refrigerator for a period of time, usually 24 hours, while the enzyme does its job.

By the way, milk shouldn't be your only source of calcium. There are several other dietary sources, including dark green leafy vegetables and oily fish with bones. (See Chapter Six: Maintaining Proper Nutrition with Lactose Intolerance for more information on the importance of calcium and how to make sure you're getting enough.)

Q: Lactase drops sound like an easy and effective way for people with lactose intolerance to continue enjoying milk—especially if they can't find commercial brands of low-lactose milk at their local groceries. What are the biggest advantages to the use of lactase drops?

A: There are many. One of the biggest is that the drops can be added to almost any kind of milk, including whole, low-fat, fat-free, chocolate, powdered, and condensed, so anyone can use the drops regardless of what kind of milk they commonly consume. In addition, commercial enzyme drops are very effective at eliminating lactose, and the more drops you add, the less lactose you'll consume. Some products claim a near 100 percent elimination after the milk has been allowed to sit in the refrigerator for at least 24 hours. Better yet, the enzyme continues to work after 24 hours, removing still more lactose from unconsumed portions.

Another benefit is the substantial convenience and savings lactase drops offer to the people who use them. For many with lactose intolerance, liquid enzyme is their only option because they are unable to find commercially produced low-lactose milk and other dairy products in their area. And when they do, they often find that such products are considerably more expensive than regular milk. By comparison, lactase drops are a better deal.

Many people also prefer the taste of milk hydrolyzed with lactase drops because it tends to be a bit sweeter than lactose-rich regular milk. This is because glucose and galactose individually are sweeter than lactose. Parents often find that their finicky children prefer milk treated with lactase over nontreated milk because hydrolized milk appeals more to their sweet-sensitive palates.

Q: Is there a downside to the use of lactase drops in making reduced-lactose milk?

A: Not many, but there are a few. For example, lactase drops should not be added to buttermilk or other cultured milk products (such as yogurt) because they have a much higher acidity level than regular milk. In addition, the enzyme drops must be refrigerated after opening to maintain effectiveness, which makes it difficult to take them with you while traveling. And, as noted earlier, the drops can cause milk to taste sweeter, which some people find difficult to swallow.

It must also be noted that while lactase drops remove nearly all of the lactose in a carton of milk if enough drops are used and the milk is allowed to sit for a sufficient length of time, they do not remove all of the lactose. There will always be a tiny amount. Most people with mild to moderate lactose intolerance will find this inconsequential, but it could still result in symptoms in individuals who suffer from extreme forms of the condition. They are a small minority, but people who fall into this category should still take note.

Q: I like the idea of using commercial reduced-lactose milk. How is it made, and what can you tell us about these products?

A: Even though commercially produced reduced-lactose milk tends to cost a little more, a growing number of people with lactose intolerance are finding it an acceptable solution to the milk conundrum (I like it, I need it—I just can't drink too much of it). In fact, manufacturers report that such products are almost three times as popular as lactase pills.

Commercial reduced-lactose milk is appealing for a wide variety of reasons. It looks like regular milk, tastes like regular milk (though perhaps a little sweeter) and, most importantly, you can drink it whenever you want, as opposed to having to wait a day or more for lactase drops to work their magic in regular milk.

The manufacture of reduced-lactose milk is pretty similar to that of regular milk, except that lactase is added during processing to lower lactose levels by 70 percent or more by the time the milk is placed on store shelves. The enzyme most typically used is produced by *K. lactis*, and is the same enzyme found in drops for home use.

One of the biggest differences between commercial lactose-reduced milk and regular milk is the way it is pasteurized. During normal pasteurization, milk is exposed to temperatures of 180°F for about 30 seconds. Lactose-reduced milk undergoes what is known as Ultra High Temperature pasteurization, which means 30 seconds at 180°F, followed by steam infusion to 290°F for two seconds and then a microorganism-killing vacuum treatment. At the completion of this process, the milk is completely free of bacteria and has a shelf life of up to 60 days. By comparison, milk that undergoes normal pasteurization has a maximum shelf life of about 12 days.

A longer shelf life has advantages for both consumers and manufacturers. Because adults with lactose intolerance typically don't drink huge amounts of milk, they don't have to worry that a carton of reduced-lactose milk will go bad before they can finish it. And manufacturers, many of them small companies, can distribute their products to a wider geographic area because their products stay fresh longer.

Unfortunately, as noted earlier, most commercial reduced-lactose milks tend to cost considerably more than regular milk. There are a number of reasons for this. First, the production of lactose-reduced milk is more costly than that of regular milk. Secondly, while popular among individuals with lactose intolerance, lactose-reduced milks don't sell nearly as well as regular milk with lactose, so manufacturers must charge a little more in order to make a profit.

Q: What kinds of reduced-lactose milk product are currently available?
A: The selection is almost as diverse as that of regular milk, though distribution may vary from region to region. Currently available, say manufacturers, are reduced-lactose whole milk, 2% and 1% low-fat milk, 1% low-fat chocolate milk, calcium-fortified milk and even 100% lactose-reduced low-fat milk. The latter product is very good news for people who cannot tolerate even the small amounts of lactose found in most commercial reduced-lactose products. However, the label of "100% lactose-reduced" is somewhat in error. Such products receive an additional dose of enzyme to eliminate still more milk sugar, but the total elimination

of lactose is almost impossible. A very, very tiny amount will always remain no matter what manufacturers do, but this minuscule amount is too small to affect the vast majority of people with even severe lactose intolerance. Some might consider this false advertising—100% should mean 100%. But state and federal packaging laws realize that absolutes are seldom possible in food processing and allow for small amounts of a given compound. For all intents and purposes, however, milk labeled 100% lactose-reduced is exactly that.

Q: Like a lot of people, I drink milk for its nutritional value—especially its calcium content. However, because I'm lactose intolerant, I can't drink very much of it. I've noticed reduced-lactose milk in the dairy section of my local grocery and would like to give it a try. Is reduced-lactose milk as nutritious as regular milk?

A: Yes. Reduced-lactose milk has the same amounts of essential nutrients as regular milk—including vitamin A, vitamin D, calcium, phosphorus, and magnesium. The only difference is that lactase is added to substantially reduce the level of lactose. We'll discuss the issue of maintaining proper nutrition with lactose intolerance in Chapter Six.

Q: Are there any other commercial lactose-reduced dairy products aside from milk? Personally, I'd love some lactose-reduced ice cream!

A: So would a lot of people with lactose intolerance. But dairy products made with lactose-reduced milk can be very difficult to find. Most manufacturers shy away from them because such products simply don't sell well enough to justify the cost. Reduced-lactose milk is a special case because milk is a common grocery item and enough people with lactose intolerance buy specialty brands to make them profitable. But the interest in related dairy products just doesn't seem to be there. At least not yet. Every now and then, however, a company will make an attempt, so keep checking the dairy section of your favorite supermarket. And if you find a reduced-lactose product that you like, tell all of your friends with lactose intolerance and write the manufacturer a letter of encouragement. Word-of-mouth support can go a long way.

In the meantime, keep in mind that being lactose intolerant doesn't necessarily mean you can never again enjoy a frozen dessert. While regular ice cream may be out of the question (unless you take a lactose pill), you can still consume frozen yogurt (most people with lactose intolerance are able to tolerate yogurt because it contains active cultures that aid digestion), Italian ices, and desserts made with soy milk instead of cow's milk.

Q: A friend recently told me that they even make special lactose-reduced milk for cats! Is that true, or was she just pulling my leg?
A: It may sound bizarre, but it's absolutely true. Ak-Pharma, the parent company of Lactaid, has released in limited markets a lactose-reduced milk treat for cats called CatSip. Don't laugh—contrary to popular belief, milk is not good for cats. Like many humans, most cats have trouble digesting lactose, and may suffer from symptoms similar to lactose intolerance when they consume fresh milk. In addition to being very low-lactose, CatSip is rich in taurine, an amino acid that is instrumental for good feline health. No other commercial milk product contains taurine, though most cat foods are for-

tified with it. CatSip can be found in many of the larger pet stores and specialty shops. For further information, check out the AkPharma website at www.akpharma. com, or call the company toll-free at 800-228-7479.

Q: My doctor has been a great help in managing my lactose intolerance. He suggested I try lactase pills so I could continue to enjoy my favorite lactose-containing foods, and they work pretty well. His most recent recommendation is capsules containing some sort of bacteria. I'm hesitant because I always thought that lactose intolerance was caused by bacteria in the intestines. Do you know what my doctor is talking about?

A: Your doctor is most likely talking about a new product from DairyCare that consists of capsules containing *Lactobacillus acidophilus* cultures, which are sometimes used to make yogurt. The concept behind the product, which as of this writing has limited distribution, is that the symptoms of lactose intolerance can be greatly reduced by replacing the intestinal bacteria which cause symptoms with another form of bacteria (*Lactobacillus acidophilus*) that produces lactase and helps digest lactose.

If the literature is to be believed, *Lactobacillus acidophilus* capsules have a number of advantages over traditional lactase pills. The biggest advantage is that, when taken as directed, the capsules provide continuous relief from the symptoms of lactose intolerance. This means that you should be able to eat lactose-containing foods whenever you want to without having to worry about the onset of symptoms. Fewer capsules are also required, so the long-term cost should be less than the use of lactase supplements.

Lactobacillus acidophilus has been added to fresh milk for a number of years, and is often recommended for people with gastrointestinal disorders—including lactose intolerance. In theory, milk fortified with the bacteria should be better tolerated by people with lactose intolerance, but there has been a lot of debate as to whether this is true. Anecdotal reports, primarily from individuals with lactose intolerance, suggest that it is not. However, there is a minority who swear by such products. It all depends on the individual. DairyCare's *Lactobacillus acidophilus* capsules will probably meet with similar results. The bottom line: It certainly couldn't hurt to give them a try.

For more information on this product, contact DairyCare via the Internet at www.dairycare.com/.

FIVE

Diseases that Mimic
Lactose Intolerance

QUENTIN WAS ABSOLUTELY CERTAIN THAT HE WAS LAC-
tose intolerant. He had the symptoms—intestinal cramping and watery diarrhea, usually after meals—and the
family history. It seemed so logical and consistent that
he didn't see how it could be anything else.

Quentin's condition began to develop shortly after he
graduated from college, and increased in severity and
frequency as the years went on. He made a self-diagnosis
early on after hearing about lactose intolerance on a television talk show, and confirmed it by reading numerous
newspaper and magazine articles on the condition.
Quentin was so confident about his diagnosis that he
never bothered to see a doctor for a breath hydrogen test
or other definitive examination. "I saw no need for it,"
says the 34-year-old postal employee. "I ate foods containing lactose and experienced symptoms of lactose intolerance. At the time, it seemed black-and-white. There
couldn't have been any other answer."

Quentin tried to manage his condition by maintaining a low-lactose diet and taking lactase pills with his meals. Sometimes they worked, but usually they didn't. When symptoms did occur, Quentin rationalized the situation by telling himself that he simply hadn't taken enough lactase to do the job, or that the foods he had consumed contained more lactose than he had anticipated.

Eventually, however, Quentin had to face the fact that his condition might be something more serious than lactose intolerance. In addition to the digestive distress he usually experienced, Quentin noticed that he was losing weight despite the fact that he ate as much as he always had. He also noticed a growing fatigue no matter how much sleep he got, as well as occasional, unexplained bouts of nausea. Fearing the worst, Quentin made an appointment with his primary care doctor for a complete medical examination.

Quentin's doctor had taken care of him for nearly a decade, but was unaware of Quentin's digestive difficulties because Quentin had never mentioned them before. As his doctor proceeded with the physical examination, Quentin explained them in detail, as well as his self-diagnosis of lactose intolerance. He also noted the weight loss, growing fatigue, and mysterious nausea.

After posing a number of questions, Quentin's primary care doctor dismissed Quentin's self-diagnosis of lactose intolerance. Though he had some of the symptoms, their frequency and timing didn't fit the pattern. Neither did Quentin's other medical problems. Realizing that Quentin needed someone with greater expertise in gastrointestinal medicine, the doctor referred him to a local gastroenterologist who specialized in inflammatory bowel disorders.

The gastroenterologist talked at length with Quentin

about his eating habits, lifestyle, and digestive problems. He asked Quentin if he had noticed any blood in his stool, or pain and bleeding from the rectum. He then asked Quentin to bring back a stool sample, and suggested he undergo a colonoscopy and other tests so he could take a closer look at Quentin's intestines. Though he knew the procedures would be uncomfortable, Quentin readily agreed. "I was terrified I had colon cancer," Quentin says now. "I thought for sure I had six months to live. At that point, I would have agreed to anything."

Happily, Quentin didn't have colon cancer. And as his primary care doctor had predicted, lactose intolerance wasn't his primary ailment, either. The colonoscopy and a barium X-ray confirmed that Quentin's actual problem was Crohn's disease, a chronic inflammation of the intestines. Though there is no cure for the disease, it can usually be controlled through medication and changes in diet and lifestyle.

"I had mixed feelings when my gastroenterologist broke the news to me," Quentin says. "I was ecstatic that I didn't have cancer, but fearful of the diagnosis of Crohn's disease because I wasn't sure what that was. Life would have been so much easier if I had simple lactose intolerance. However, my doctor worked closely with me to bring the condition under control and manage it effectively. I still get flare-ups, some of which are rather severe, but not nearly as often as I used to. The most important thing is that I have a definitive diagnosis of my problem, and I know how to treat it. As long as I'm careful, I should be okay."

Quentin's story illustrates well the fact that, when it comes to digestive disorders, things aren't always as they seem. Lactose intolerance is a very common problem, but a wide variety of conditions can mimic its symptoms. Many people, like Quentin, incorrectly self-diagnose their problem based on a minimal understanding of lactose intolerance but never see a doctor for a definitive answer until other symptoms unrelated to lactose intolerance come into play.

In this chapter, we'll discuss the various intestinal conditions whose symptoms often mimic lactose intolerance, including irritable bowel syndrome, Crohn's disease, and ulcerative colitis, with special emphasis on their symptoms, diagnosis, and treatment.

Q: The symptoms of lactose intolerance seem so clear-cut. How could it be confused with other medical disorders?

A: The symptoms of lactose intolerance are clear-cut, but they have to be analyzed in a specific context. If you drink a large glass of whole milk and an hour later find yourself experiencing incapacitating cramps, bloating, and diarrhea, the likely diagnosis is lactose intolerance—especially if these symptoms occur only after you consume lactose-rich foods. However, numerous intestinal diseases can also present these symptoms (and others), and may also manifest themselves following meals, so it's easy to see how such disorders could be confused with lactose intolerance.

The frequency with which certain intestinal disorders are mistaken for lactose intolerance illustrates three things: (1) the importance of seeing a doctor at the first onset of symptoms, (2) the importance of getting a breath hydrogen test or other definitive exam to confirm a suspected diagnosis of lactose intolerance, and (3) the potential harm that can come from self-diagnosing your problem without the input of a doctor. Now you know why doctors are so reluctant to make a diagnosis based only on a patient's description of symptoms; armchair docs are quite often wrong.

Q: How common is lactose intolerance compared to ailments with similar symptoms?

A: In the big picture, lactose intolerance is far and away the most common digestive disorder of its type—far more common than those disorders that can mimic its symptoms. You'll recall from Chapter One that some authorities call lactose intolerance the most common genetic condition in the world, afflicting tens of millions, perhaps hundreds of millions worldwide. By comparison, disorders such as Crohn's disease, ulcerative colitis, and irritable bowel syndrome are relatively uncommon, though far from rare. Ulcerative colitis (including ulcerative proctitis) has an incidence of approximately 6 to 8 cases per 100,000 people and estimated prevalence of 70 to 150 cases per 100,000 people. The incidence of Crohn's disease is somewhat smaller, with an estimated 2 cases per 100,000 people and an estimated prevalence of 20 to 40 cases per 100,000 population.

Q: Relatively speaking, how serious is lactose intolerance compared to the many disorders that can mimic its symptoms?

A: While lactose intolerance can be an aggravating problem to those who have it, it's a minor inconvenience when compared to many of the more serious problems that can affect the gastrointestinal tract. In severe cases of ulcerative colitis or Crohn's disease, for example, the surgical removal of portions of the intestines may be required to bring relief from symptoms. Treatment that dramatic is almost never required for simple lactose intolerance. So consider yourself extremely lucky if all you have to do to prevent symptoms is take lactase pills or make sure you eat one scoop of ice cream instead of two.

Of course, this in no way is meant to diminish the impact and importance of lactose intolerance. It can be a very serious condition, resulting in extremely painful symptoms and major changes in lifestyle. But in the big picture, things could be considerably worse.

Q: For almost a year I thought I was lactose intolerant, but when I finally had a breath hydrogen test, it came back negative. My doctor performed a number of other tests and told me I had inflammatory bowel disease. What is this, and how does it affect the intestines?

A: Inflammatory bowel disease is an umbrella term for a handful of ailments that adversely affect the lining of the intestines, resulting in painful and aggravating symptoms. Doctors are unsure what causes these disorders, nor is there a definitive test for their diagnosis. As a result, doctors usually confirm inflammatory bowel disease through a differential diagnosis that gradually eliminates all other potential disorders.

Inflammatory bowel disease (not to be confused with irritable bowel syndrome, which is a separate ailment discussed on page 134) is typically divided into two major groups—chronic nonspecific ulcerative colitis and Crohn's disease. Inflammatory bowel disease was first described in 1932 and localized to areas of the ileum. However, researchers later discovered that the disease could also affect other areas of the gastrointestinal tract, including the buccal mucosa (mucous membrane), esophagus, stomach, duodenum, jejunum, and colon.

Crohn's disease of the small intestine is also known

as regional enteritis, and a similar inflammatory problem may also occur in the colon, either alone or with involvement of the small intestine. In the majority of cases, this specific form of inflammatory bowel disease is distinguishable from ulcerative colitis and is also known as Crohn's disease of the colon.

Symptoms of Crohn's disease include diarrhea, abdominal pain, diminished appetite, weight loss, weakness, fatigue, nausea, and vomiting. Symptoms of ulcerative colitis include severe and bloody diarrhea, abdominal pain, poor appetite, weight loss, mild fever, anemia, and loss of body fluids.

Ulcerative colitis and Crohn's disease share a similar development and symptoms, but are considered distinct medical disorders. They afflict men and women in similar numbers, but are more common in whites than in blacks or Asians. They also have an increased incidence (up to sixfold) in Jews compared to non-Jews. Onset of both disorders typically occurs in young adulthood, between the ages of 15 and 35, but it can afflict people of any age. Researchers believe there is either a genetic or an environmental connection (possibly both) because studies have shown that between 2 and 5 percent of people with either condition have one or more close relatives who are similarly afflicted.

Q: I understand that doctors don't know what causes the various forms of inflammatory bowel disease, but do they have any theories?
A: There are numerous theories regarding the potential cause of the varied forms of inflammatory bowel disease, though more research is needed before a definitive answer can be determined. Common theories include:

- **Genetics**. As noted earlier, people with inflammatory bowel disease are likely to have a close family member who is also affected (a medical phenomenon known as "clustering"). In addition, the condition is known to hit certain ethnic populations more commonly than others, and studies have found an increased incidence of Crohn's disease in monozygotic twins. All of this suggests a strong genetic predisposition to the development of the disease, say some researchers. However, as of this writing, the ongoing search for a specific genetic marker has revealed little.

- **Infection**. Because of the inflammatory nature of inflammatory bowel disease, some researchers believe it may be caused by an infectious agent, perhaps viral, bacterial or fungal. But to date, no specific agents have been identified or isolated. Infectious agents are known to produce acute, or isolated, episodes of colitis or ileitis, but there is no evidence that these agents play any role in chronic inflammatory disease.

- **Immune response.** Some researchers believe that there may be an autoimmune mechanism associated with the development of inflammatory bowel disease because of the type of disorders that often accompany it, such as arthritis. As a result, it has also been theorized that therapeutic agents commonly prescribed for the treatment of inflammatory bowel disease, such as glucocorticoids (a type of steroid), work by easing that autoimmune mechanism. However, researchers have been unable to verify with certainty an autoimmune connection, and this theory is receiving less and less acceptance within the research community.

- **Psychological factors.** Could psychological stressors or a certain personality type play a role in the development of inflammatory bowel disease? Some researchers believe there may be a connection. It's commonly known that ulcerative colitis and Crohn's disease both flare up in association with major psychological stresses such as death of a family member, loss of a job, divorce, or other negative emotional situations. As a result, some researchers speculate that patients with inflammatory bowel disease have a specific characteristic personality that makes them susceptible to emotional stresses that in turn may precipitate or worsen symptoms. While there's little clinical evidence linking emotional factors to the onset or cause of inflammatory bowel disease, it's common knowledge that a chronic condition of unknown origin which afflicts people at the height of life can result in feelings of anger, anxiety, and even depression. Such reactions are important factors in modifying the course of inflammatory bowel disorders as well as their response to therapy.

Q: What happens to the body as a result of inflammatory bowel disease? How does it affect the intestines to cause telltale symptoms?

A: What you're asking about is what's known in medicine as the pathology of the disease—the course it takes and how it affects various organs and body systems. It's somewhat complicated, but I'll try to make it as easy to understand as possible.

As its name suggests, inflammatory bowel disease is a serious inflammation of the intestines. In ulcerative colitis, this inflammatory reaction primarily involves the colonic mucosa. The colon appears ulcerated, hyperemic (congested with blood) and usually hemorrhagic, hence the common symptom of blood in the stool. What's unique about this inflammation is that it is uniform and continuous throughout the colon, with no areas of normal mucosa. In about 95 percent of cases, the rectum is involved. When the entire colon is affected, the inflammation may extend a few inches into the terminal ileum (the end portion of the ileum), a condition commonly referred to as "backwash ileitis."

The inflammation that characterizes ulcerative colitis is often quite severe and damaging, affecting the ability of the colon's surface cells to do their job. Chronic bouts of inflammation often result in the development of fibrosis, although unlike in Crohn's disease, deeper layers of the bowel beneath the submucosa are usually unaffected. In severe ulcerative colitis, the bowel wall may become extremely thin, the mucosa stripped and inflammation extending to the serosa (the thin membrane lining the intestine), resulting in intestinal widening and perforation.

Crohn's disease, while similar in many ways to ulcerative colitis, has a number of distinct characteristics. For example, chronic inflammation extends through all layers of the intestinal wall and usually involves the small intestine's supporting membrane (known as the mesentery) as well as regional lymph nodes.

The very early effects of Crohn's disease are not well understood because surgery is rarely performed during this stage of the ailment so researchers can't get a close-up look. Many patients at this stage of the disease develop regional intestinal inflammation (known as enteritis), but a surprisingly high number recover completely. The cause of these sudden flare-ups has yet to be determined, though some patients have been shown to be infected with *Yersinia enterocolitica*, a microorganism capable of triggering a self-limiting form of inflammatory ileitis.

If the condition becomes chronic, as is often the case, its progress becomes fairly typical. The bowel appears greatly thickened and leathery, and the interior passage becomes increasingly narrow. This characteristic constriction can occur in any segment of the intestine and may be linked to varying degrees of intestinal blockage. The mesentery appears thickened, fatty, and often extends over the serosal surface of the bowel in tiny, fingerlike projections.

The appearance of the mucosa, or the intestine's interior surface tissue, can vary dramatically according to the stage or severity of the disease. If the disease is relatively mild, it may appear normal and healthy—especially in comparison to ulcerative colitis. In severe or advanced cases, however, the mucosa often has a nodular look that somewhat resembles cobblestones—the result of submucosal thickening and mucosal ulceration. These ulcerations, or sores, can penetrate into the submucosa (the deeper layers of the intestinal wall) and harden to form abscesses (localized collections of pus surrounded by inflamed tissue). The abscesses can spread to other areas to form fistulas (small, pipelike abscesses) and fissures (a break or ulceration where skin and mucous membrane join, most commonly found in the anus and around the anal area).

There are a number of other pathological differences between ulcerative colitis and Crohn's disease. For example, while ulcerative colitis usually affects the entire colon, Crohn's disease typically shows inflamed segments separated by areas of normal, healthy bowel tissue. In addition, the rectum is spared in nearly half of all cases of Crohn's disease of the colon whereas with ulcerative colitis, the rectum is almost always affected. And fistulas, which are common in Crohn's disease, are almost never seen in ulcerative colitis.

Despite these and other differences, ulcerative colitis and Crohn's disease are quite similar in pathology and symptoms and thus are often frustratingly difficult to differentiate in many patients, doctors say. The microscopic identification by a rectal or coloscopic biopsy of mucosa showing granulomas (nodules of tissue that form as a reaction to chronic inflammation) is one of the most definitive ways of distinguishing Crohn's disease from similar kinds of inflammatory bowel disease because they do not occur as a normal part of ulcerative colitis. However, while the detection of granulomas can be helpful, it is the chronic inflammation involving all the layers of the intestinal wall which is the most identifiable characteristic of Crohn's disease. In approximately 10 to 20 percent of patients, though, it may be impossible to make an accurate distinction between ulcerative colitis and Crohn's disease of the colon.

Q: Is Crohn's disease uniform in its attack on the intestines, or does it affect certain parts more than others?

A: According to gastroenterologists, the distribution of Crohn's is fairly uniform. Studies have found that approximately 30 percent of cases involve the small intestine (usually the terminal ileum) without colonic disease; 30 percent involve only the colon, and 40 percent will have ileocolic involvement usually of the ileum and right colon. However, in a small number of patients—most commonly children and teenagers—there may be widespread and extensive ulceration of the jejunum and ileum.

Q: Earlier, you briefly mentioned the most common symptoms of ulcerative colitis and Crohn's disease. Could you please elaborate on the characteristic symptoms of both disorders?

A: Yes. The primary symptoms of ulcerative colitis are bloody diarrhea and abdominal pain. If the disease is mild, there may be one or two semiformed stools containing little blood and no other bodily symptoms. But if the disease is severe, it may result in frequent watery diarrhea containing blood and pus, severe cramps, dehydration (from the diarrhea), anemia (from blood loss), fever, and weight loss. If the rectum is very involved, a patient may complain of an urgent need to defecate that is frequently unsuccessful (a phenomenon known medically as tenesmus). Sometimes the intestinal symptoms of ulcerative colitis are overshadowed by more systemic complaints, such as fever or weight loss.

Severe cases of ulcerative colitis can also result in systemic symptoms that seemingly have little to do with the gastrointestinal tract, including arthritis, skin changes, evidence of liver disease, tachycardia (rapid heartbeat) and low blood pressure when sitting or lying down (postural hypotension). The findings of laboratory tests are often nonspecific and usually just reflect the degree and severity of bleeding and inflammation. Anemia, for example, may reflect chronic disease and an iron deficiency from long-term blood loss. And electrolyte abnormalities, which are detected by a blood test, may reflect chronic diarrhea.

The progression of ulcerative colitis is unpredictable, though the majority of patients experience a relapse within one year of the first attack, reflecting the recurrent or chronic nature of the disease. But sometimes there can be extended periods of remission during which the patient experiences minimal symptoms or none at all. And then there are patients who experience a quick progression of the disease, with escalating severity of symptoms. According to doctors, an estimated 85 percent of patients with ulcerative colitis will have a mild to moderate form of the disease and can be successfully managed without hospitalization. In the remaining 15 percent of patients, the disease progresses quickly and severely, affecting the entire colon and other parts of the body. These patients can develop a dangerous distention of the colon called toxic megacolon (a massive distention of the large intestine). They are at high risk for perforation of the colon and are often considered medical and surgical emergencies.

The primary clinical symptoms of Crohn's disease are fever, abdominal pain, and diarrhea (usually without blood), as well as generalized fatigue and, occasionally, associated weight loss. If the colon is involved, diarrhea and pain are the most common symptoms. Rectal bleeding is much less common than with ulcerative colitis, though there may be anorectal complications such as fistulas, fissures, and perirectal abscesses (pus-filled lesions around the anal area), all of which can be extremely painful. Distention of the colon may occur if there is extensive colonic involvement, but because the colon typically thickens with Crohn's disease, this is observed much more commonly in ulcerative colitis.

As with ulcerative colitis, other bodily changes such as arthritis may afflict patients with Crohn's disease, though they are more likely to occur with Crohn's disease of the colon rather than the small intestine. However, involvement of the small intestine may result in additional symptoms. This form of Crohn's disease occurs most commonly in young adults who may have had earlier complaints of fatigue, variable weight loss, frequent bouts of diarrhea, and pain or discomfort in the lower right area of the abdomen. Low-grade fever, anorexia, nausea, and vomiting may also be present. Not surprisingly, many people with rapid-onset Crohn's disease are first thought to be suffering from acute appendicitis. The types of symptoms and their severity can have a broad range, and may be influenced by factors such as age and overall health.

The complications of Crohn's disease can be specific to a particular area of the intestines, and result from intestinal inflammation and involvement of nearby tissue and organs. One of the most common localized complications is intestinal obstruction, which typically is caused by acute inflammation and swelling of the involved intestinal segment. It afflicts between 20 and 30 percent of patients during the course of the disease. Fistula formation is another common complication of Crohn's disease of the colon, and frequently occurs between connected segments of the intestine. In a large number of patients, the first manifestation of Crohn's disease may be the presence of persistent rectal fissures, a perirectal abscess, or a rectal fistula.

Crohn's disease may also involve the stomach and duodenum, with symptoms suggesting a peptic ulcer. In rare cases, as the disease progresses it may cause chronic scarring of the gastric outlet (the opening between the stomach and the duodenum) or a duodenal obstruction.

Another potential complication associated with Crohn's disease is increased risk of cancer of the small intestine and colon, most typically in patients who have had the disease for a long time. However, though the risk of developing a malignancy is statistically increased as the disease goes on, the complication is relatively uncommon when compared to the frequency of cancer related to ulcerative colitis. Gallstones may also develop as result of damage to the ileum and subsequent bile salt malabsorption.

Q: What kinds of tests are available for the diagnosis of inflammatory bowel disease?
A: Unlike lactose intolerance, there are no tests that definitively diagnose the various forms of inflammatory bowel disease; doctors usually make a diagnosis based on the patient's symptoms and medical history. However, sigmoidoscopy, colonoscopy, and radiologic studies can be extremely helpful in confirming certain indicating factors.

Sigmoidoscopy and colonoscopy are essentially the same procedure. The difference is that a sigmoidoscopy looks only at the sigmoid colon (the area nearest the rectum), while a colonoscopy looks deeper into the large intestine and thus may require a sedative or anesthesia. In both procedures, a tube is inserted through the anus and gently guided into the terminal ileum. With the help of a tiny videocamera, the doctor can then see for himself the condition of the colon, whether there is any obvious ulceration or other tissue changes, and how serious they are. If necessary, the doctor can also use the device to snip off a tiny piece of tissue (a procedure known as a biopsy) for microscopic examination and testing.

Most gastroenterologists recommend a colonoscopy or sigmoidoscopy for all patients complaining of abdominal pain, chronic diarrhea, and/or rectal bleeding, which are strong indicators of inflammatory bowel disease. In ulcerative colitis, the findings of a colonoscopy can include continous inflammation, ulcerations, and bleeding of the intestinal lining. Indicators of Crohn's disease can include tiny ulcerations and/or deep fissures, as well as stretches of healthy intestinal tissue between inflamed patches. Pseudopolyps (harmless nodules that shouldn't be confused with potentially cancerous polyps), swelling, and strictures may also be seen in Crohn's disease as well as in ulcerative colitis (pseudopolyps are seen more frequently in ulcerative colitis, however).

A radiologic evaluation of the bowel can also provide important information in the diagnosis of inflammatory bowel disease, say gastrointestinal specialists. For example, a barium X ray (in which the colon is filled with an opaque liquid using an enema and then X-rayed) can help diagnose ulcerative colitis by revealing the extent of the disease and defining associated features such as ulcerations, stricture, pseudopolyps, or cancer. The earliest feature seen with ulcerative colitis as a result of irritation of the intestinal tissue is incomplete filling caused by a lack of distention (enlargement) of the colon. A barium X ray may also reveal fine ulcerations along the contour of the bowel. These ulcerations usually become deeper and more pronounced as the disease progresses.

In addition, a barium X ray can help diagnose Crohn's disease by distinguishing the condition from ulcerative colitis. Features characteristic of Crohn's disease include little involvement of the rectum (known medically as rectal sparing) and the detection of ulcerations occurring on irregular intestinal nodules. The test may also show irregular thickening of the intestinal wall that can lead to the formation of strictures, or abnormal narrowing of the intestine. In 10 to 15 percent of cases, Crohn's disease may uniformly affect the entire colon, making it difficult for doctors to differentiate it from ulcerative colitis.

A barium X ray of the colon can be very beneficial in diagnosing inflammatory bowel disease and confirming the specific type, but it's not for everyone. For example, the procedure can actually make things worse in patients with severe forms of colitis, and trigger dangerous widening, or dilatation, of the colon. It can also be extremely painful in patients with severe intestinal ulceration (imagine dragging a long piece of plastic along an open sore). Other tests that are used in the diagnosis of inflammatory bowel disease include an upper gastrointestinal (GI) series, in which a barium X ray is taken of the esophagus, stomach, and duodenum, and a computed tomography (CT) scan of the abdomen to assess complications such as abscesses, fistulas, and obstruction.

Gastroenterologists use all of the above when making a differential diagnosis of inflammatory bowel disease. Making a differential diagnosis, you'll remember, is similar to being a detective—all potential causes are gradually ruled out until only the real cause remains. Because of the wide array of symptoms that characterize bowel disease and the large number of potential culprits, a differential diagnosis is often the only way a doctor can accurately confirm the cause of a patient's symptoms.

The focus of the differential diagnosis is largely determined by the patient's obvious symptoms. Rectal bleeding, for example, could be caused by a wide variety of problems, including hemorrhoids, colonic tumors, diverticulitis, or intestinal ulcerations. That's why a colonoscopy can be so advantageous—by taking a look at the intestinal lining, the doctor can quickly eliminate a large number of potential causes.

Q: How is inflammatory bowel disease typically treated?

A: In the majority of cases of mild to moderate inflammatory bowel disease, symptoms can be controlled with medication and certain lifestyle changes. Surgery is reserved for very severe cases, or the onset of potentially life-threatening complications.

Treatment for ulcerative colitis and Crohn's disease is relatively similar, though there can be substantial differences between the two in areas such as response to drug therapy, complications, and prognosis following surgery.

Medical therapy for ulcerative colitis, once it has been definitively diagnosed, depends on the severity of the disease. Mild ulcerative colitis can often be treated on an outpatient basis, while severe cases may require a stay in the hospital. The goal of therapy is to control the inflammatory process and replace nutritional losses, so patients may receive fluids to correct electrolyte imbalances and blood transfusions to correct anemia. Medications to control diarrhea may also be prescribed, but these are used sparingly because of the risk of causing colonic distention and toxic megacolon. Patients may also receive nutritional supplements if the condition has resulted in mild malnutrition caused by poor absorption during digestion. Supplementation is often given intravenously in cases in which anything consumed by mouth stimulates the colon, a common problem in severe cases of ulcerative colitis.

The drugs most commonly prescribed for the treatment of ulcerative colitis include anti-inflammatory agents such as sulfasalazine (Azulfidine) to prevent recurrence. In very severe cases in which general treatment appears ineffective, doctors may prescribe a stronger anti-inflammatory in the form of glucocorticoids (steroidal anti-inflammatories such as Prednisone)—considered the "big gun" in the treatment of ulcerative colitis.

Once ulcerative colitis has been brought under control through medical therapy, patients may also benefit from psychotherapy. Ulcerative colitis certainly is not considered a psychological disorder, but many patients become resentful of the disease and the impact it has on their lives and may fall into a state of depression. This is especially common among children, adolescents, and the elderly. In these cases, psychotherapy, combined with aggressive medical treatment, can help patients resolve emotional issues, cope better with the disease, and get on with their lives.

Unfortunately, a significant number of ulcerative colitis cases progress to the point where medical treatment is no longer effective or the patient's life is in jeopardy because of related complications. In such cases, the surgical removal of the entire colon (a procedure known as a colectomy) may be necessary. Gastroenterologists say that approximately 20 to 25 percent of all people with ulcerative colitis eventually require a colectomy over the course of the disease. It's a major medical and life event and not one to be considered lightly by either the patient or his doctor, but the majority of ulcerative colitis patients who undergo a colectomy report that their lives are dramatically improved as a result. People who undergo a complete removal of the colon will require a procedure known as a colostomy, in which the remaining end of the bowel is brought up through the skin, creating what's known as a stoma. Fecal material is collected in a disposable pouch that attaches to the skin around the stoma. Specialists known as enterostomal therapists work with such patients regarding the care and maintenance of colostomies and related procedures.

The treatment for Crohn's disease is similar in many ways to that of ulcerative colitis, with the drug sulfasalazine most commonly used to reduce inflammation of the colonic tissue. Glucocorticoids are also useful, researchers report, though they tend to work better on Crohn's disease of the small intestine than Crohn's disease of the colon.

Though medical intervention is usually successful during the initial attack of Crohn's colitis, many patients continue to suffer from recurrent flare-ups and related complications. Medication is often helpful in managing these problems, though patients must be closely monitored by their doctors. As with ulcerative colitis, many patients with Crohn's disease experience nutritional disorders that require supplementation, either by mouth or intravenously.

There are also some steps patients can take on their own to ease the effects of a flare-up of Crohn's disease. If you have diarrhea, for example, it usually helps to avoid foods that have a laxative effect, such as raw fruits and vegetables and concentrated fruit juices. It's also a good idea to give your intestines a rest by avoiding solid foods for a day or so after the flare-up. Instead, drink clear liquids throughout the day to prevent dehydration. Rehydrating beverages such as Gatorade are best because they contain many of the compounds your body needs during this problem time. When the bout of diarrhea is over, slowly return to your normal eating habits by consuming small but frequent meals. Abdominal cramps can often be alleviated by placing a heating pad set on low or a hot-water bottle on the painful area.

Surgical intervention is often required for Crohn's disease, though usually it is reserved as a last-ditch treatment for complications rather than a primary form of therapy. According to gastroenterologists, an estimated 70 percent of patients will need at least one operation during the course of their disease. The most common reasons are for persistent or fixed narrowing of the bowel; obstruction of the bowel; the formation of fistulas on the bladder, vagina, or skin; persistent anal fistulas or abscesses; and toxic dilatation or perforation of the colon. Unlike ulcerative colitis, in which surgery is usually a cure, patients with Crohn's disease often continue to have recurrences of the disease following the surgical removal of portions of the bowel. But despite these recurrences, most patients can expect a dramatic improvement in their health.

Q: Now that we understand inflammatory bowel disease and how it is treated, what's the prognosis for those who have it? Do most live long, active lives?
A: Yes. Thanks to effective management techniques and innovative new treatments, the majority of people with inflammatory bowel disease do relatively well. With acute ulcerative colitis, which is characterized by occasional flare-ups rather than a chronic condition, improved therapeutic techniques result in a remission in nearly 90 percent of patients. However, prognosis is not as good when the entire colon is involved, when onset occurs over the age of 60, or when toxic megacolon occurs.

The long-term prognosis for chronic ulcerative colitis is more difficult to predict because of the variable nature of the disease and improvements in therapy. In general, patients with chronic ulcerative colitis do well when treated aggressively, though 75 percent will still experience relapses and, as noted earlier, between 20 and 25 percent will eventually require a colectomy.

According to gastroenterologists, the long-term prognosis for Crohn's disease is not quite as good as for ulcerative colitis. The disease doesn't respond as well to medical therapy with time, and nearly two-thirds of patients develop complications requiring surgery at some point in their lives.

Q: I'm 28 and have lived with ulcerative colitis for several years. I've managed to keep it under control fairly well with the help of my doctor, and I feel pretty good. My husband and I would like to have a baby, but I'm concerned that my condition could cause problems. Is it safe for me to become pregnant?

A: Most likely, yes. But you should still talk with your doctor just to make sure.

In the past, doctors often discouraged women with ulcerative colitis and Crohn's disease from having children for fear that the diseases would impact on their pregnancy and their unborn children. However, more recent studies have found that pregnancy is rarely affected by coexistent inflammatory bowel disease, and that there is no increase in stillbirths or premature deliveries when compared to the general population.

You should know, however, that pregnancy triggers flare-ups of the disease in about 50 percent of women with inactive colitis. Most colitis attacks are clustered in the first trimester of pregnancy and following birth. Treatment for the disease during pregnancy is pretty much the same as at any other time, with the most common therapy being sulfasalazine to ease inflammation.

As for the health of your child—don't worry. Studies have found that sulfasalazine is perfectly safe for pregnant women and their unborn babies.

Women with active colitis or Crohn's disease are encouraged to bring their conditions under control before attempting to become pregnant in order to ensure the healthiest physical and emotional environment for pregnancy.

Q: A good friend of mind thought she was lactose intolerant, but later was told she has something called irritable bowel syndrome. Is this the same thing as inflammatory bowel disease?

A: No. Though they sound alike and may have similar symptoms, irritable bowel syndrome (IBS) and inflammatory bowel disease (IBD) are two different disorders. According to medical authorities, irritable bowel syndrome is the most common gastrointestinal disease seen by doctors, and though it's not fatal, it can cause its victims—and the doctors who treat them—a lot of aggravation and frustration.

Irritable bowel syndrome comes in three different forms. Patients with so-called spastic colitis usually complain of chronic abdominal pain and constipation. A second variation is characterized by chronic intermittent diarrhea—often without pain. And a third form has features of the previous two with alternating diarrhea and constipation.

Indications of psychological disturbances, including depression, hysteria, and obsessive-compulsive traits, are sometimes seen in patients with irritable bowel syndrome, and psychological stress can make symptoms of the disorder worse.

Irritable bowel syndrome is most often seen in young

or middle-aged adults, and afflicts women far more often than men (some studies suggest a four-to-one ratio). The most common feature is a history of chronic constipation, diarrhea, or both occurring at specific intervals over a period of months or years. The diarrhea is usually worse in the morning and after breakfast (which could encourage some people to make an erroneous self-diagnosis of lactose intolerance), and relatively rare in the evening or at night. Very often the diarrhea will occur for extended periods, then suddenly disappear for no apparent reason.

A diagnosis of irritable bowel syndrome is based on a number of medical observations. Foremost is the chronic intermittent nature of symptoms without the additional signs of physical illness that often characterize inflammatory bowel disease. Doctors also look for a link between symptoms and environmental or emotional stress. However, a differential diagnosis may be required to rule out other conditions.

Q: How is irritable bowel syndrome typically treated?
A: With a lot of patience, say doctors. Irritable bowel syndrome is a chronic condition and can't be cured, but symptoms can usually be relieved. However, it often takes time.

The psychological components of irritable bowel syndrome are just as important as the physical. Patients often fear that their condition will lead to inflammatory bowel disease or colon cancer, and should be reassured by their doctors that this rarely is the case. Patients should also be encouraged to adapt to symptoms in order to minimize the impact on their lifestyle and be made aware that emotional stress can cause symptoms to flare up or worsen. And lastly, patients should be informed that certain foods, especially those that are extremely spicy or have a high fat content, can trigger symptoms in sensitive individuals.

Irritable bowel syndrome is typically managed with drug therapy designed to alter the patient's specific abnormal colon function. Increased fiber in the diet, for example, is often an effective treatment for constipation, and chronic watery stools can usually be treated with antidiarrhea medications. However, no specific drug or dietary regimen is effective in all patients, so a little trial and error may be necessary.

Q: I was recently diagnosed with Crohn's disease, and was devastated by the news. Thankfully, my doctor is encouraging and is working hard to help me manage my condition. What can I do to help myself?

A: There's plenty you can do, doctors say. Foremost, always be aware that symptoms can come back at any time. This awareness will help prevent you from feeling depressed or fearful when a recurrence does happen. In addition, you may find it helpful to:

- Maintain a positive attitude. Learn to live with your condition and try not to let it get you down.
- Learn some relaxation techniques such as mental imaging, deep breathing, and muscle relaxation exercises. They can help you control stress and anxiety.
- Make sure your family and friends are aware of your condition and what you must do to keep it under control. An understanding support group can

be very beneficial in preventing stressful or anxious situations that could lead to a recurrence.

- Eat well, but if necessary, avoid foods that could irritate your digestive system, such as spicy dishes and raw fruits and vegetables. Talk with your doctor about the possible need for dietary supplements such as calcium or a multivitamin tablet.
- Try to exercise regularly, even if it's just a brisk walk around the block. Thirty minutes of vigorous exercise at least three times a week can do wonders for both your physical and mental health.
- Make sure you get enough sleep.
- Listen to your doctor and follow her advice and instruction when it comes to your condition. If she starts to talk to you in "medical-ese," don't hesitate to ask her to repeat the information in more understandable terms.

Q: After decades of enjoying dairy products, I noticed what seemed to be the onset of lactose intolerance. However, after conducting a number of tests (including a breath hydrogen test) my doctor informed me that my symptoms were actually being caused by my diabetes, which I've controlled with insulin for more than decade. How can diabetes produce many of the same symptoms as lactose intolerance?

A: The occurrence of chronic diarrhea and other symptoms similar to those seen in lactose intolerance is well documented among people with long-standing diabetes mellitus. That's because diabetes can affect a large number of body systems—including the gastrointestinal tract.

Doctors theorize that many cases of diabetes-related diarrhea involve the autonomic nervous system with degenerative changes in the sympathetic and parasympathetic nerves. (The sympathetic and parasympathetic divisions of the nervous system control the motor functions of the heart, lungs, intestines, glands, and other internal organs, and the smooth muscles, blood vessels, and lymph vessels.) An overabundance of bacteria in the small intestine may also contribute to the condition.

Diabetic diarrhea is fairly consistent in its presentation, doctors say. It usually occurs in patients in which diabetes developed at a young age and was difficult to control. Men are afflicted far more often than women. Upon examination, there are usually signs of autonomic neuropathy (a disease of the part of the nervous system responsible for certain "uncontrollable" functions such as breathing and blood pressure) including low blood pressure, impotence, and bladder problems. Related vascular disease may also be noted.

If the problem is related to bacterial overgrowth, antibiotics are usually the treatment of choice. In addition, the drug clonidine has proved effective in patients with severe diarrhea that doesn't respond well to dietary measures or other drug therapy such as anticholinergics.

I'm assuming your doctor has given you a thorough examination and is treating your condition effectively. But if you continue to have diarrhea and other symptoms, talk with your doctor about alternative therapies.

Q: Is it possible to have inflammatory bowel disease and lactose intolerance at the same time?
A: Yes. Lactose intolerance and other malabsorption disorders are a fairly common secondary complaint among people with Crohn's disease and can wreak havoc with the intestinal lining and dramatically affect its ability to produce lactase, which is needed for the

digestion of lactose. As a result, people with inflammatory bowel disease often find it useful to take lactase supplements during meals to aid the digestion of milk sugar in the foods they eat.

If you have inflammatory bowel disease and suspect you may also have lactose intolerance, talk to your doctor about performing a breath hydrogen test to confirm your suspicions. If the test is positive, your doctor can help you devise a dietary plan that will help reduce symptoms and ensure you're receiving adequate nutrition.

Q: Can lactose intolerance lead to inflammatory bowel disease or irritable bowel syndrome?
A: No. Lactose intolerance by itself does not lead to further medical problems in the gastrointestinal system, although, as noted earlier, it can be a secondary complaint among people who already have inflammatory bowel disease or irritable bowel syndrome. And in those individuals, awareness of lactose intolerance can sometimes bring additional relief.

In a recent study published in the *Journal of Clinical Gastroenterology*, researchers tested patients with irritable bowel syndrome for lactose intolerance to see if identifying lactose intolerance and changing dietary habits would ease symptoms of irritable bowel. A little more than three and a half years later, the researchers interviewed the test subjects again and found that they showed no significant differences in abdominal pain, altered bowel habits, bloating or distention, mucus, and relief with defecation. However, "all of the lactose-maldigesting IBS subjects reported that identifying lactose maldigestion influenced their awareness of lactose-symptom relationships and brought some improvement,'' the researchers noted.

The moral: Even though lactose intolerance does not cause irritable bowel syndrome, awareness of lactose intolerance and an effort to maintain a low-lactose diet may help ease certain symptoms and make life a little more tolerable for people with IBS.

Common Causes of Chronic Diarrhea

Diarrhea, gas, and painful bloating are all common indicators of lactose intolerance. But as we've seen in this chapter, lactose intolerance is not the only possible cause; a wide array of diseases, medical disorders and conditions can also result in one or more similar symptoms. They include:

Inflammatory disorders
Infectious parasites, bacteria, viruses, and fungi
Crohn's disease (regional enteritis)
Ischemic bowel disease (ischemic colitis)
Diverticulitis
Proctocolitis
Ulcerative colitis

Tumors and unusual tissue growth
Colorectal cancer
Polyposis
Villous adenoma
Intestinal lymphoma
Zollinger-Ellison syndrome
Vasoactive intestinal peptide syndromes

Malabsorption disorders
    Chronic pancreatitis
    Pancreatic carcinoma
    Biliary obstruction
    Bacterial overgrowth syndromes
    Celiac sprue
    Tropical sprue
    Whipple's disease
    Lymphangiectasia
    Hypogammaglobulinemia
    Eosinophilic gastroenteritis
    Amyloidosis

The result of outside influences (medical treatment, lifestyle and others)
    Radiation enteritis
    Irritable bowel syndrome
    Drug-induced
    Poison/chemicals
    Laxative abuse
    Postoperative
    Gastrectomy
    Jejunoileal bypass
    Short-bowel syndrome
    Ileocolostomy
    Ileal resection
    Pancreatectomy

Metabolic/systemic disorders
    Hyperthyroidism
    Hypoparathyroidism
    Adrenal insufficiency
    Uremia
    Connective tissue diseases

Metabolic/system disorders (con't)
  Cystic fibrosis
  Mastocytosis
  Porphyria
  Cystinuria
  Fabry's disease

Miscellaneous causes
  Food allergies
  Chronic, severe congestive heart failure
  AIDS

(List adapted from *Practical Strategies in Outpatient Medicine, Second Edition* by Brendan M. Reilly, M.D.; W.B. Saunders Company, 1991, table 15-13, p. 866; used by permission.)

SIX

Maintaining Proper Nutrition with Lactose Intolerance

AGNES GREW UP IN A HOUSEHOLD WHERE MILK AND other dairy foods were considered the foundation of good nutrition. Her mother, a registered nurse, constantly emphasized the importance of eating right, and made certain that Agnes and her two older brothers always drank a large glass of whole milk with every meal. "To my mom, milk was the perfect food," recalls Agnes, now 30. "She saw it as a way of making sure that my brothers and I got all of the essential nutrients our growing bodies needed."

As might be expected, Agnes inherited her mother's obsession with good nutrition. She continued to make milk and other dairy products a mainstay of her diet after she moved away from home to attend college, and later when she moved to Chicago to take a job as a paralegal with a prominent law firm.

It was a few years after she transferred to Chicago that Agnes began to develop aggravating and often painful digestive problems, including gas, bloating, and watery diarrhea. "It quickly became apparent that dairy products were the cause of my condition," Agnes says. "At first my symptoms were relatively minor, and I thought I could live with them. But within a year they were occurring every day and getting consistently worse, so I simply stopped eating dairy. Within a week, my symptoms were almost gone. I thought I had my problem licked."

Agnes tried to eat right on her new, dairy-free regimen but didn't always succeed. Fast food was a big part of her daily diet, as was microwavable "meals for one." Junk food filled her pantry, and soft drinks replaced her beloved milk. When Agnes finally saw her doctor for an insurance-related physical examination, he expressed alarm at her lifestyle, diet, and suspected nutritional deficiencies.

"My doctor lectured me for nearly half an hour," Agnes notes. "He explained how my dietary regimen—or lack of one—could impact on my health, and emphasized the importance of calcium, vitamin D, and other nutrients in preventing osteoporosis and related conditions in women. I told him that too much dairy makes me sick, so he showed me how to determine my dairy threshold. He also gave me a long list of alternate sources of essential vitamins and minerals, many of which I had never considered before."

Agnes took her doctor's advice to heart and started eating with better nutrition in mind. She now eats much less fast food and junk food, and consumes at least a small amount of milk or other dairy products every day—always mindful that she doesn't exceed her established limits. Agnes also makes sure her home-cooked meals contain plenty of calcium-rich nondairy foods such as green leafy vegetables, yogurt, legumes, and sea-food (particularly canned fish with bones, such as her-ring and salmon), and she takes calcium supplements and a multivitamin tablet every day.

"I have an aunt with severe osteoporosis, so I know how it can ravage the body," Agnes states. "I don't want that to happen to me. Dairy products are an excel-lent source of calcium and other essential nutrients, but I can't eat as much of them as I used to. So I make up for it in other ways. Just because a person is lactose intolerant doesn't mean she can't eat well and maintain proper nutrition. It may require a little more effort, but it's definitely worth it."

Indeed, poor nutrition is one of the biggest concerns among people who cannot consume as much lactose-containing food as they used to. Rather than looking for nutritional substitutes, often they simply avoid dairy products, and thus jeopardize their health. This is a par-ticularly important problem among lactose-intolerant women because of the risk of bone-weakening osteo-porosis and related disorders. In this chapter, we will discuss the nutritional importance of dairy products, the Recommended Daily Allowance (RDA) of calcium and other nutrients, and alternative sources for these essential vitamins and minerals.

Q: Throughout childhood I was told to drink my milk so I would grow up big and strong. But no one really explained why milk and other dairy products are so important to good nutrition. What am I missing if I don't have them in my diet?

A: A lot, say nutrition experts. Milk, cheese, and other dairy products contain a genuine wealth of essential vi-tamins and minerals—the building blocks of good nutrition and thus of good health during every stage of life. The most important nutrient found in dairy products is calcium, which is one of the most abundant minerals in our bodies and necessary for the building and mainte- nance of strong bones and teeth, as well as several im- portant body functions. But that's not all. Milk also contains many other essential nutrients including vita- mins A, B_6, B_{12}, C, D, and E, thiamin (vitamin B_1), riboflavin (vitamin B_2), niacin, iron, phosphorus, mag- nesium, zinc, protein, carbohydrates, fat, and calories. Some of these nutrients are more important than others and supplied in greater amounts than others, but all of them are vital to our physical and mental well-being. Without them, important body systems would work less efficiently, and we would get sick more often and more severely.

People with lactose intolerance often avoid all dairy products because they fear developing symptoms. How- ever, doctors say most individuals with the condition can consume at least small amounts of dairy products, and are encouraged to do so (within their personal limits) in order to maintain proper nutrition. The use of lactase supplements, as discussed in Chapter Four, can often be beneficial in this endeavor because they allow people with lactose intolerance to consume even greater quan- tities of healthful dairy products without developing symptoms. People who have the condition should also talk with their doctors about their possible need for nu- tritional supplements, even if it's just a daily multivita- min or mineral supplement tablet.

Q: Why is calcium so important to our bones and teeth? And in what other ways does it benefit the body?

A: If we consumed no calcium at all, our bones would find it extremely difficult to grow and repair themselves. The reason: Bone is living tissue that is continually being broken down and rebuilt via a hormone-triggered process known as remodeling. This is how our bones grow and maintain themselves for most of our lives, and it requires a lot of calcium for the job to be done right.

As might be expected, bones grow most quickly throughout childhood and adolescence. More than one-third of our total adult bone mass develops between the ages of 9 and 18, doctors note, as old bone is replaced by new bone approximately every three months. During our 20s, bone growth increases by approximately 15 percent, and peak bone mass—the time at which our bones are at their strongest—typically occurs between the ages of 25 and 35. After that, bone mass slowly diminishes (the process of dissolution occurs faster than the rate of new bone creation) and our bones begin to lose their strength. This explains why older people are more prone to bone fractures than younger people.

In addition to building and maintaining healthy bones, calcium plays an important role in helping blood clot and the heart muscle to contract. So important is calcium to this process that an imbalance in either direction can have a direct impact on our health.

Ideally, we should get all the calcium our bodies need from the foods we eat—primarily dairy products, which are literally packed with the mineral (an 8-ounce glass of milk contains more than 35 percent of the RDA for calcium). But when we don't consume enough calcium via our diet to meet our bodies' needs, our bodies must look elsewhere for it. This usually means that the body leaches calcium from the bones (where 99 percent of our calcium deposits are stored) to maintain a consistent supply in the bloodstream. The result: Weakened bones and increased risk of fractures.

Q: How much calcium does the body need through each stage of life? Is more required during certain ages than others?

A: Yes. The recommended daily allowance (RDA) for calcium as set by government health-and-nutrition experts fluctuates quite a bit depending on age and gender. Everyone needs the mineral, but women require considerably more than men, especially if they are pregnant, nursing, or menopausal. The minimum daily allowance of calcium for anyone over 18 is 800 milligrams, but you definitely should consume more than that if possible.

There has been quite a bit of discussion in recent years regarding the recommended daily allowance of calcium. Many experts, including a consensus development panel convened by the National Institutes of Health in 1994, believe that several age groups and populations would benefit greatly from an increased RDA of this essential mineral, and most nutritionists and dieticians now support the new RDA totals. The suggested RDA for calcium is as follows:

Children and young adults:

- 0–6 months—400 milligrams
- 6–12 months—600 milligrams
- 1–10 years—800–1,200 milligrams (formerly 1,200 milligrams)
- 11–24 years—1,200–1,500 milligrams (formerly 1,200 milligrams)

Adult women:

- Below 24 years, pregnant or breast-feeding—1,500 milligrams (formerly 1,200 milligrams)
- 25 and over, pregnant or breast-feeding—1,200 milligrams
- 25–49 years—1,000 milligrams (formerly 800 milligrams)
- 50–64 years, taking estrogen—1,000 milligrams (formerly 800 milligrams)
- 50–64 years, not taking estrogen—1,500 milligrams (formerly 800 milligrams)
- 65 and older—1,500 milligrams (formerly 800 milligrams)

Adult men:

- 25–64 years—1,000 milligrams (formerly 800 milligrams)
- 65 and older—1,500 milligrams (formerly 800 milligrams)

Q: Why do women need so much more calcium than men?
A: Because bone mass in women is greatly affected by hormones, specifically estrogen, and greater amounts of calcium are required throughout a woman's life to make sure that her bones will continue to be strong after menopause. Women's bones tend to be less dense anyway, but the decrease in estrogen that typically accompanies menopause can result in a condition known as osteoporosis, which is characterized by a potentially dangerous loss of bone density and strength.

Women who are pregnant also need additional amounts of calcium because a growing fetus pulls calcium from the mother during development. In other words, the mother is consuming calcium for two. A baby's calcium requirements are relatively small in the beginning, but teeth and bones require the mineral when they start to form around 4 to 6 weeks after conception. By the 25th week of pregnancy, when a baby's bone growth is at its highest, a woman's calcium requirements will have almost doubled. Breast-feeding also increases a woman's calcium demands as her body works to produce sufficient amounts of nourishing milk for her new baby.

Q: Is it true that calcium may help alleviate the symptoms of premenstrual syndrome?

A: It appears so. According to researchers at St. Luke's-Roosevelt Hospital Center in New York, symptoms of premenstrual syndrome (PMS), such as bloating, cramping, mood swings, and breast tenderness, may be an indicator of a calcium deficiency that could lead to weak and brittle bones later in life. Certain' women may not absorb or utilize calcium properly, says lead study author Dr. Susan Thys-Jacobs. As a result, they develop symptoms that are associated with PMS but which actually may be a warning that not enough calcium is reaching their bones and they should increase their intake. PMS sufferers who took 1,200 milligrams of calcium carbonate daily for three months reduced their symptoms by almost 48 percent.

Q: I'm lactose intolerant, and my doctor has warned me that if I don't get started taking calcium supplements I'm going to have a greatly increased risk of osteoporosis by the time I reach menopause.

Could you tell us a little bit more about this condition?

A: Sure. Osteoporosis is a very common disease afflicting an estimated 25 million people in the United States—more than 80 percent of them women. As noted earlier, its most common symptoms are loss of bone density and reduced bone strength, and it is the most frequent cause of bone fractures in postmenopausal women and the elderly.

Osteoporosis can be a very debilitating disorder. Related fractures can occur in almost any bone, doctors say, but the most frequent location is the spinal column. Bone loss to the spinal column occurs quite quickly following menopause, and many women are surprised to learn that they received a painful spinal compression fracture through a very simple act, such as bending over to put away groceries. Changes to the spinal column can also result in reduced height as the spine compresses and a curvature of the spine commonly known as ''dowager's hump.''

Gerontologists (doctors who deal with the problems associated with aging) report that fractures to the hip and wrist are also very common among individuals with osteoporosis, and such breaks can be quite devastating. Hip fractures among the elderly, studies show, are one of the most serious health problems in the United States because they are associated with more deaths, greater disability and higher medical costs than all other osteoporosis-related problems put together. An estimated 20 percent of the elderly die within a year of breaking their hips, and of those who survive, fewer than half return to their previous level of activity even after undergoing physical therapy.

A number of factors are involved in the potential development of osteoporosis. They include:

- **Age.** Denser bones can delay the onset of osteoporosis, but gradual bone loss is an inevitable part of aging. Women can take preventive measures, however, by consuming plenty of calcium throughout their lives.
- **Gender.** Because women's bones are less dense by nature, and because menopause tends to promote a loss of bone mass, osteoporosis is nearly eight times more common in women than men. But that's not to say that men don't need to keep an eye on their calcium intake—they do. Osteoporosis may be less common in men, but its effects can be equally devastating.
- **Early menopause.** Gynecologists warn that women who enter menopause early as a result of disease or the surgical removal of the ovaries are at risk of early onset of osteoporosis.
- **Ethnic background.** White and Asian women are at greater risk of developing osteoporosis than African-American women. The reason: African-American women typically have a bone mass that is approximately 10 percent greater than that of white and Asian women.
- **Lack of weight-bearing exercise.** This is one of the few factors women can influence, doctors say. Weight-bearing exercises such as walking, aerobics, and racquet sports promote stronger muscle mass. As a result, women who do not exercise regularly are at greater risk of developing osteoporosis. Researchers have found that astronauts who spend a great deal of time in weightlessness come home

with a noticeable reduction in bone mass—proof that weight-bearing exercise (defined as activities that force bones to work against gravity) really is helpful.

- **Body weight.** Women who are thin and small-boned are at greater risk of osteoporosis, even at a young age. This is especially true of small, athletic women who exercise so strenuously that they stop menstruating.

- **Heredity.** A family history of osteoporosis (either diagnosed or evidenced by telltale symptoms such as frequent broken bones or curvature of the spine) should put women on alert that they are at increased risk of developing the disease.

- **Alcohol and tobacco consumption.** Women who smoke and drink heavily typically have weaker bones than women who don't engage in these harmful habits. The reason: Smoking inhibits the absorption of calcium, and drinking affects bone formation. If you engage in one or both of these habits, think seriously about quitting.

- **Disease and medications.** Osteoporosis can be a side effect of certain diseases, such as hyperthyroidism, rheumatoid arthritis, kidney disease, and certain types of cancer. It can also result from the long-term use of certain medications such as thyroid hormones, steroids, and anticonvulsants. If you have a chronic disease or must take medication for extended periods, consult with your doctor about the risk of osteoporosis and how it can be prevented.

Q: Osteoporosis sounds like an inevitable part of aging for most women. Can it be prevented?

A: Yes. Osteoporosis can often be prevented, even if a woman has a number of the risk factors listed above, but it takes a lot of hard work and dedication. According to doctors, if a woman's bones reach their maximum density, or mass, by the time she turns 30, and if she makes a conscious and concerted effort to curb the rate of natural bone loss later in life by getting enough calcium and other nutrients, she can reduce her risk of osteoporosis to almost zero.

Obviously, the prevention of osteoporosis is not something that a woman should consider for the first time when she hits menopause. For the best results, adequate calcium consumption should be started in childhood and maintained throughout adulthood. A panel of experts convened to research this issue concluded that maximum calcium intake is most important from childhood through age 25 or so, because that's when the bones grow their fastest. Other peak periods of consumption include the months immediately following menopause (when estrogen levels usually plummet) and during the later years. Regular exercise can also play an important role in keeping the disorder at bay—as well as benefiting one's overall physical and mental well-being.

Talk with your doctor if you're unsure whether you're getting sufficient amounts of calcium. She can gauge your consumption and offer some tips on how to get more if necessary.

Q: I'm lactose intolerant, but I want to make sure I'm getting enough calcium in my diet. What are some of the best sources of this essential mineral besides dairy products?

A: There are several excellent sources of calcium, including a variety of nondairy foods and over-the-counter supplements. A combination of both can usually guarantee that you're getting optimum levels for your age and needs.

Dairy products, as most people know, are packed with calcium. An 8-ounce glass of milk contains approximately 300 milligrams of calcium—one-fourth the amount recommended for growing children and young adults. But this doesn't do you any good if you're severely lactose intolerant (unless you're willing to use lactase supplements to help you digest it). Luckily, there are quite a few alternative dietary sources for this very important mineral. Many vegetables, for example, contain high levels of calcium. One spear of raw broccoli contains 72 milligrams of calcium, while one cup of chopped, cooked broccoli contains 354 milligrams. One cup of steamed, fresh collards contains 357 milligrams of calcium, and an equal amount of kale offers another 179 milligrams. Other calcium-rich vegetables include artichokes, asparagus, mustard greens, okra, turnip greens, brussels sprouts, cabbages, leeks, parsley, rutabagas, carrots, cauliflower, green peas, lettuce, radishes, and tomatoes.

Men and women who are concerned about calcium are advised to consume only small amounts of vegetables with high levels of oxalic and phytic acids because they can actually inhibit calcium absorption. These include beets and beet greens, eggplant, green beans, onions, rhubarb, spinach, corn, kidney beans, lima beans, pinto beans, soybeans, brown rice, and wild rice. These vegetables shouldn't be avoided completely because many of them contain small amounts of calcium as well as greater amounts of equally important nutrients. Just be sure not to make them the focus of your meal.

Many kinds of fish and other seafood are also rich in

calcium. Canned fish with soft bones, such as herring, mackerel, sardines, and salmon, contain very high amounts—3 ounces of salmon contains 167 milligrams of calcium, and an equal amount of sardines contains a whopping 370 milligrams. Nutrition experts say that clams, oysters, and shrimp are also good sources of calcium.

Realizing the importance of calcium in the American diet, many food manufacturers are now offering products fortified with extra calcium. The most common are fortified breads and flours, but a close look at food labels may reveal others.

Individuals with lactose intolerance should also look to yogurt and tofu as sources of extra calcium. Yogurt, while definitely a dairy product, is usually well tolerated by people with lactose intolerance because it contains active cultures that aid digestion. One cup of plain, low-fat yogurt contains 415 milligrams of calcium, and an equal amount of fruit-flavored, low-fat yogurt has approximately 345 milligrams. Tofu, which is made from soy, is another excellent source. One medium-sized square of tofu contains about 100 milligrams of calcium, and levels can be even higher when tofu is processed with calcium sulfate.

Calcium supplements can also be useful in guaranteeing that you consume sufficient amounts of calcium—but they shouldn't be your only source. Several different types of calcium supplements can be found on store shelves, but most nutrition experts recommend either calcium citrate or calcium carbonate. Both forms have specific advantages. Calcium citrate makes a little more calcium available to the body, and clinical studies have found that it also causes fewer side effects such as constipation, digestive problems, and kidney stones. Calcium carbonate, on the other hand, contains the highest percentage of absorbable calcium gluconate. If you have trouble swallowing pills, consider calcium-rich chewable or liquid antacids. Many brands are now being touted as effective sources of calcium.

Calcium supplements to avoid include "chelated" calcium tablets (which tend to cost more and have little else to offer over regular supplements) and calcium supplements with magnesium (this is usually unnecessary because most people get sufficient amounts of magnesium through the foods they eat). While it's true that vitamin D is necessary for the effective absorption of calcium, most people get sufficient amounts through their diet and exposure to sunlight. However, certain groups of people, such as seniors and postmenopausal women, may need to take calcium and vitamin D supplements. Consult your doctor if you think you may need to take one or both of these supplements. Most nutrition authorities also recommend that you stay away from "natural" supplements such as dolomite or bone meal (which is produced from ground animal bone) because they may contain potentially harmful substances such as arsenic, lead, and mercury. There is a debate on this issue, but it's wise to be cautious.

Calcium supplements are generally most effective when taken with meals because stomach acid aids in their absorption. It is also recommended that calcium supplements be taken over the course of the day rather than all at once. The best-absorbed products will note on their labels that they meet U.S. Pharmacopoeia (USP) standards, but you can also test them at home by dropping a tablet in a small glass of white vinegar. If it doesn't dissolve completely within a half hour, it won't absorb well in your stomach either.

Q: How do I determine how much of a particular calcium supplement I should take? Sometimes product labels can be a bit confusing regarding specific amounts.

A: Remember: Calcium supplements shouldn't be your sole source of the mineral—you should still get the biggest percentage from the foods you eat. That's why they call them supplements. As for specific amounts of absorbable calcium, look for the words *elemental calcium* on the label. That's how much will actually be absorbed by your body. A warning should go off in your head if the label doesn't provide this information or doesn't distinguish between the total amount of calcium carbonate or calcium citrate and elemental calcium. You may be getting less elemental calcium than you need.

As for the amount you should take each day, first determine what your specific recommended daily allowance is based on your age and other factors (if you are pregnant, breast-feeding, or menopausal, for example) and make a determination from there. Let's assume that you're 30 years old, not pregnant, a nonsmoker, and in otherwise good health. Your RDA of calcium is 1,000 milligrams per day. If the supplements you're taking provide, say, 300 milligrams of elemental calcium, then two or three a day (600 to 900 milligrams) should be more than enough—assuming you are also eating sufficient amounts of calcium-rich foods.

If you have additional factors to consider, such as a chronic illness or the need for daily medication, check with your doctor to determine how much calcium you should take and the form that's best for you.

Q: Consuming sufficient calcium doesn't seem too difficult. Are most Americans getting enough of the

mineral to ward off osteoporosis and other disorders?

A: Sadly, no. According to national health care officials, millions of Americans aren't getting enough calcium to prevent the development of osteoporosis later in life. This was confirmed by a recent national survey in which it was discovered that the average daily intake of calcium ranges from 530 milligrams among middle-aged women to a high of 1,179 milligrams among teenage boys. On average, very few American women are getting the recommended 800 milligrams or more per day of calcium, even though they need it the most.

Several factors are responsible for this dilemma. Hectic schedules at home and at work often prevent women from eating well or exercising regularly. But even when women do sit down to a home-cooked meal, it's often lacking in calcium-rich foods and/or is made up of foods that can affect the body's ability to absorb calcium. The two most common calcium absorption inhibitors are caffeine and salt. Researchers have concluded that just two cups of caffeinated coffee a day over the course of a woman's lifetime can result in a noticeable decrease in bone density because coffee and other caffeine-containing drinks such as cola and cocoa stimulate the loss of calcium through the kidneys and intestines. Salt also pulls quite a bit of calcium into the kidneys, where it is excreted in urine. The more salt you add to your food, the greater the calcium loss.

In addition, many women engage in the types of life-style habits that can greatly affect the body's ability to absorb and use calcium, such as smoking and alcohol consumption.

Q: I recently saw a calcium supplement that contained calcium lactate. Since I'm lactose intolerant, could taking this particular type of supplement result in symptoms?

A: No. The only thing that can cause symptoms in people with lactose intolerance is lactose—and calcium lactate supplements contain none. It's just another form of calcium that happens to have a similar-sounding name. It's an effective supplement, but other varieties, such as calcium carbonate, usually contain substantially higher percentages of elemental calcium.

Q: Can you take too much calcium? Is the mineral dangerous in high doses?

A: Most people don't get enough calcium, so too much is rarely a concern. But the answer to your question is yes, it is possible to consume too much calcium, and problems could result if you do.

According to the 1994 National Institutes of Health consensus panel discussed earlier, calcium supplementation in adults is considered safe in amounts up to 2,000 milligrams a day. That amount is even higher in children and adolescents—2,500 milligrams a day—because those are the most crucial years for bone formation. Studies have shown that such high amounts of calcium produce no side effects in young people, and may reduce the risk of bone fractures later in life by as much as 50 percent.

In adults, excessively high amounts of calcium (usually through the overuse of supplements) can cause a number of serious health problems, including painful kidney stones from calcium salts building up in the kidneys.

Early warning signs of calcium oversupplementation include dry mouth, constipation, drowsiness, headache, and chronic fatigue or weakness. If overuse continues, an individual could also experience confusion, nausea, vomiting, depression, hypertension, bone or muscle pain, photosensitivity, and an irregular heartbeat. If you are taking calcium supplements and notice more than a few of these signs, stop taking the supplements and see your doctor immediately—especially if you feel a noticeable change in your heartbeat. Calcium overdose is rare, but supplement users should be aware of the symptoms.

Q: You mentioned earlier that vitamin D is required for the absorption of calcium. Should people with lactose intolerance be concerned about getting sufficient amounts of this nutrient?

A: The amount of vitamin D you consume is not as big a concern as the amount of calcium, but it is still something to be aware of because vitamin D is a very important nutrient. It increases the amount of calcium and phosphorus the body absorbs in the small intestines; controls the growth, hardening, and repair of bone tissue; is vital to the normal growth and development of bones, cartilage, and teeth in children; and prevents rickets, a unique deficiency disorder that results in malformed bones and teeth in children and thin, brittle bones in adults.

Q: Could you please give us more information on vitamin D? I'd like to know the RDA for this nutrient, as well as how I can make sure I'm getting enough.

A: There are two forms of vitamin D—ergocalciferol (which can be found in certain foods) and cholecalciferol (which the body manufactures naturally when exposed to sunlight). Vitamin D is fat-soluble, meaning excess amounts are stored in fat tissue rather than excreted out of the body, and thus can be dangerous if taken in large amounts over a long period of time.

The recommended daily allowance for vitamin D is fairly standard. Children should receive about 800 International Units (IU) of vitamin D through age 18 because it helps build strong bones and teeth. From ages 19 through 22, the amount can be reduced to 600 IU daily. For adults age 23 and older, the requirement is 400 IU of vitamin D daily.

Women who are pregnant or breast-feeding are encouraged to take an extra 400 IU of vitamin D daily to aid the absorption of the additional calcium they also should be consuming. Both nutrients are essential to a baby's growth and development. However, do not exceed this amount, nutrition experts warn, because too much vitamin D during pregnancy can result in fetal abnormalities. Men and women over age 55 may also need additional amounts of vitamin D to help in their fight against osteoporosis. This is especially true of post-menopausal women.

There are several good dietary sources of vitamin D. Milk and other dairy products are often fortified with the nutrient, but again, this does you little good if you're lactose intolerant. Instead, adequate amounts of vitamin D can usually be obtained by consuming regular portions of certain oily fish with bones, such as herring, mackerel, salmon, and sardines. Cod-liver and halibut-liver oils also contain high amounts of this nutrient. If you're not into seafood, you can get plenty of vitamin D from dark green leafy vegetables, liver, wheat germ, whole grains, dried beans, nuts, and seeds. Vitamin D supplements are also available for those who need them.

Q: What kinds of problems can result from taking too much vitamin D?

A: Most vitamins are safe even in high doses, but vitamin D is not one of them. Megadosing is strongly discouraged because, as noted, vitamin D is stored in the body rather than flushed out, and toxicity can result if you take too much.

Large amounts taken over a long period can result in a dangerous buildup of calcium in the blood (a medical condition known as hypercalcemia) that can damage the kidneys and cause various soft tissues to become hard, particularly in the lungs, stomach, blood vessels, and joints. Too much vitamin D can also cause kidney stones, constipation, and abdominal pain. See your doctor immediately if you are taking vitamin D supplements and experience any of these symptoms.

Q: Is it true that calcium and vitamin D can play a role in reducing the risk of certain cancers?

A: It appears so. Population analysis studies have found a distinct correlation between low levels of calcium and vitamin D and higher rates of breast and colon cancer. Some researchers speculate that calcium binds bile and fatty acids to reduce irritation to the lining of the large intestine and impede the growth of cancer cells. There is also some evidence that vitamin D itself has cancer-fighting properties, though the exact mechanism remains a mystery.

Interestingly, geographic region appears to play an instrumental role in the development of these cancers because exposure to sunlight causes the body to produce vitamin D, researchers add. Breast and colon cancer are noticeably less common in sunny areas such as south Florida than in northern regions, where exposure to sun-

light is low (especially in the winter) and where tall
buildings leave people in the shadows all day.

**Q: Because I'm extremely lactose intolerant, I try to
maintain a relatively low-lactose, nondairy diet. I
take calcium and other nutritional supplements,
but my doctor warned that my dietary regimen
could result in dangerously low levels of protein if
I wasn't careful. Should I be concerned?**

A: Possibly. Proteins are an essential nutrient—they are
the basic building blocks for every cell in our body—
and dairy products are a common source, so you could
be at risk of a protein deficiency if you're not filling the
void with other protein-rich foods such as meat, poultry,
seafood, or grains and legumes, for example. Certain
types of vegetarian diets or low-protein weight-loss reg-
imens can also result in a potential deficiency, but this
is actually a relatively rare problem in the United States
because meat is still such a common dietary staple.

Proteins are made up of amino acids, most of which
are manufactured by our bodies. However, nine important amino acids can be obtained only from the foods
we eat, so it's important that we maintain a balanced
diet. Certain populations need more protein than others,
such as infants, children, the elderly, and pregnant or
breast-feeding women. Too little protein can result in
stunted growth in children, as well as a lack of energy
and reduced immunological protection. If protein levels
drop too far, the body is forced to leach the nutrient from
muscle in other tissue, resulting in emaciation. This is a
common problem in countries where food sources are
often limited.

The recommended daily allowance for protein is just
0.8 g/kg of body weight a day, but most Americans con-

sume far more than that in their daily diet. Good sources of dietary protein include meat (lean red meat, poultry, or seafood), beans, grains, yogurt, and tofu.

Q: Does a strict vegetarian diet provide sufficient amounts of protein?

A: Yes and no. Plants can be an excellent source of protein, but unlike animal proteins, which are considered "complete," vegetable sources are often lacking in one or more of the nine essential amino acids and must be consumed in combination to ensure that your body is getting all it needs to stay healthy. Luckily, this isn't that difficult—many of our favorite ethnic dishes are perfect examples of healthful plant protein combinations, such as lentils and rice, hummus (a mixture of chickpeas and sesame seeds), and tortillas and beans. For optimum nutrition, you should combine grains (rice, corn, wheat, oats, barley, buckwheat) with legumes (lentils, sprouts, kidney beans, lima beans, black-eyed peas, peanuts, split peas).

As Americans increasingly embrace the foods of other cultures, a growing array of tasty, protein-rich products can now be found on our grocery shelves. Most are easy to prepare (simply follow the directions on the package) and offer a pleasant change from the usual "steak and potatoes." They include:

- **Amaranth.** Looking quite a bit like golden poppy seeds, this grain has a crunchy, porridgelike texture when cooked. It tastes like corn and makes a great breakfast food.
- **Bulgur.** Made of cooked, dried, and crushed wheat, bulgur has a delicious nutty taste and makes a terrific rice substitute. Best of all, it's very nutritious

and has the same food value as whole wheat.
- **Couscous.** This very popular Middle Eastern delicacy has really caught on in the United States. It is made from finely cracked wheat and has the same texture as rice.
- **Millet.** This round grain is often used as a yummy base for chili and other dishes. It's easy to prepare and quite nutritious.
- **Roasted buckwheat groats.** Also known as kasha, these pyramid-shaped grain slivers are used in a wide variety of Eastern European dishes as well as in cereals. They're a nice alternative when you're tired of the same old grain products.
- **Tofu.** Made from soy milk, this curd product has been a nutritious, low-calorie source of protein in East Asia for more than 2,000 years. Relatively flavorless by itself, it's great when seasoned and can be found in a wide array of tasty Asian dishes, including soups.

The items listed above are just the tip of the iceberg when it comes to alternative grains. Check out the grain and bean sections of your local grocery or health food store for more protein-rich products.

Q: Is it possible to consume too much protein? And if so, what kind of health problems could result?
A: Like all nutrients, protein is vital to our good health—but it's possible to overdo it. Those most at risk are bodybuilders and other athletes who erroneously believe that extra protein equals extra muscle, and thus a better physique. A wide array of "muscle building" products containing amino acids and protein can be found in health food stores, but most people don't need

them (even athletes) and they can cause more harm than good if misused, nutrition experts warn. The reason is simple: The body cannot store unused protein. Excess protein manufactures fat or is converted into energy. The waste products from this complicated chemical conversion are passed from the body in urine, which can place a dangerous strain on the kidneys and the liver.

Remember: The RDA for protein is just 0.8 g/kg of body weight a day for most adults, and that's usually easy to achieve through your diet. Consult your doctor before taking protein supplements.

Q: Are there any other essential nutrients that people who consume little dairy should be concerned about?

A: There are a few. One of the most important is phosphorus, which is second to calcium as the most plentiful mineral in the human body. Phosphorus is essential for proper bone growth and maintenance, and can be found in every cell. It is also instrumental to every chemical reaction that occurs in the body, and helps various tissues and systems utilize vitamins, fats, carbohydrates, proteins, and other nutrients. In addition, phosphorus stimulates muscle contractions, supports cell division and growth, and promotes the transmission of nerve impulses.

The recommended daily allowance of phosphorus is 800 milligrams for most adults. Women who are pregnant or breast-feeding need an additional 400 milligrams daily to ensure optimum fetal growth and development. However, women who are pregnant or breast-feeding should consult with their doctor before taking phosphorus supplements—and they should never take more than the recommended daily allowance. The RDA for children is 240 milligrams for infants up to 6 months, 360 milligrams for ages 6 to 12 months, 800 milligrams for ages 1 to 10 years, and 1,200 milligrams for ages 11 to 17 years—a period of rapid bone growth and development.

Too little phosphorus in our diets can result in a variety of health problems including weight loss, fatigue, anemia, arthritis, stunted bone development, bone pain, tooth decay, and gum disease. Thankfully, the mineral has several dietary sources. Milk and milk products are excellent sources of phosphorus, but if you can't tolerate large amounts of dairy, pack your meals with lean red meat, calves' liver, poultry, and seafood, including tuna, canned sardines, and scallops. Other good sources of phosphorus include dark green leafy vegetables, eggs, almonds, peanuts, dried beans, peas, soybeans, pumpkin seeds, sunflower seeds, and whole-grain products. Phosphorus supplements can also be found at most grocery and health food stores. But again, talk with your doctor before taking additional amounts of this important mineral. You may be getting sufficient levels from the foods you eat.

Q: Is phosphorus dangerous in large amounts?

A: Phosphorus is a nontoxic nutrient, and there is little evidence that problems can result from taking more than the recommended amount each day. However, pregnant and breast-feeding women are encouraged not to take megadoses of the mineral as a precaution.

In a related issue, however, problems can occur when taking potassium phosphate supplements, which are often prescribed as a treatment for kidney stones. Side effects associated with potassium phosphate supplements (usually caused by potassium salts contained in the supplements) include shortness of breath, seizures, and irregular heartbeat. Common warning signs that you may be headed for a serious adverse reaction include headache, abdominal pain, joint pain, bone pain, confusion, diarrhea, muscle cramps, swelling in the feet and legs, numbness or tingling in the hands and feet, and reduced urine output. If you are on potassium phosphate supplements and notice any of the above, you should call your doctor immediately.

Q: I told a good friend of mine who is a nutrition counselor that I was on a low-lactose diet that included few dairy products, and she suggested I take supplements that included riboflavin. What is riboflavin and why is it so important?

A: Riboflavin is a water-soluble nutrient that also goes by the name of vitamin B_2. It is found in milk and other dairy products, and people with lactose intolerance could find themselves deficient if they don't get riboflavin from other dietary sources or commercial supplements.

Riboflavin is an important nutrient. It helps the body grow and develop, maintains the health of the mucous membranes and helps protect the skin, eyes and nervous system. Some researchers speculate that riboflavin also improves iron absorption within the body because iron and riboflavin deficiencies are often seen at the same time. In addition, riboflavin has a number of medical uses, particularly in the treatment of stomach and liver disorders, infections, burns, and alcoholism.

Although riboflavin is an essential nutrient, the RDA for riboflavin is actually pretty low. The suggested RDA for riboflavin is as follows:

Infants and children:

- 6–12 months—0.6 milligrams
- 1–3 years—0.8 milligrams
- 4–6 years—1.0 milligrams
- 7–10 years—1.4 milligrams

Males:

- 11–14 years—1.6 milligrams
- 15–22 years—1.7 milligrams
- 23–50 years—1.6 milligrams
- 51 years and older—1.4 milligrams

Females:

- 11–22 years—1.3 milligrams
- 23 years and older—1.2 milligrams
- Pregnant women require an additional 0.3 milligrams
- Breast-feeding women require an additional 0.5 milligrams

Nutrition authorities say that milk is the best source of riboflavin—one quart contains more of the nutrient than most people need in a day. Other adequate dietary sources include yogurt, chicken, leafy green vegetables, organ meats such as liver, cereal, bread, and wheat germ. Riboflavin is also included in most multivitamin supplements.

Q: Is it possible to take too much riboflavin? Could any health problems result if you do?
A: Riboflavin is completely safe and nontoxic, even in quantities far greater than the recommended daily allowance. Because it's water-soluble, excess amounts of ri-

boflavin are flushed from the body in urine. The only potential side effect from taking too much riboflavin is darkened urine, which is completely harmless.

Q: The typical American diet seems to have more wrong with it than right. What kinds of cuisine do dieticians recommend for people with lactose intolerance who want to make sure they're getting sufficient amounts of calcium and other nutrients?

A: You're right, the traditional American diet isn't as healthful as it could be. According to government nutrition experts, we still place too much emphasis on red meat and fatty, fried foods and not enough emphasis on grain products and fresh vegetables and fruit—items that should make up the largest portion of our daily diet. Bottom line: The average American consumes too many empty calories and not enough essential nutrients, resulting in obesity and an increased risk of heart disease and stroke.

The sad part is that eating for health doesn't have to be a chore. By merely redirecting the focus of their diets, most Americans could eat more nutritionally and prevent the onset of a number of chronic health conditions. A few tips:

- Eat more poultry and fish and less red meat. When cooking chicken, remove the skin. And when you do eat red meat, make sure it's a lean cut. Remove all fat before consuming.
- Make vegetables and fruit a part of every meal.
- Avoid fried foods. Instead, have meat, poultry, or fish broiled or baked. And instead of french fries, try a baked potato or fresh garden salad.

- Reduce the amount of salt in your diet. Replace it with other spices.
- Drink more water and fresh fruit juice and fewer empty-calorie soft drinks.
- Eat smaller portions. Some people find that it helps to use a smaller plate.
- Never shop on an empty stomach.
- Try to exercise a minimum of three times a week.

People with lactose intolerance should also consider various foreign fare. Most Asian cuisines, such as Chinese, Japanese, Korean, and Thai, are also quite nutritious and receive high marks from dieticians. Asian cuisine is rich in healthful vegetables, poultry, and seafood, and very few recipes use milk or other dairy products because of the high incidence of lactose intolerance among Asians. Instead, soy milk and tofu are often substituted for dairy. Another nice thing about Asian cuisine is that it offers a lot from which to choose. You could eat Chinese, Japanese, Thai, or Korean every day for a month and never have the same dish twice. It also appeals to a wide range of palates—from the very conservative to the very daring.

Q: Is a kosher diet also beneficial for people with lactose intolerance?

A: It can be. A kosher diet can be quite nutritious, but it's even more useful in avoiding foods that could trigger symptoms of lactose intolerance. According to Jewish dietary law, there must be a strict separation of meat (which includes poultry) and milk, both in preparation and presentation. They cannot be eaten at the same meals or on the same plate. This can be very helpful in identifying processed foods that do not have milk products in them, and avoiding those that do, since foods that meet the strict definition of kosher are usually clearly labeled. For people with lactose intolerance, the word to look for is *pareve* (also spelled *parve*). This is the indication of a "neutral" food that is completely free of both milk and meat. We'll discuss kosher diet and pareve foods in greater detail in Chapter Seven: Tips for Tolerating Lactose Intolerance.

Q: As someone with lactose intolerance, I worry about nutrition. However, I'd rather not bother my doctor with my concerns. Is there someone else who could give me some sound advice on eating right while maintaining a low-lactose diet?

A: You shouldn't worry about "bothering" your doctor with your nutrition questions. Yours is a legitimate concern and your doctor should be able to offer quite a bit of valuable advice on the subject. But if you'd still rather look elsewhere for nutrition information, you might want to consult a registered dietician (look in your local yellow pages under "Dieticians," or ask your doctor for a recommendation). There are more than 60,000 registered dieticians nationwide, and many larger medical practices have one or more on staff. In order to become a registered dietician, a person must receive at least a four-year degree in dietetics or nutrition and a 900-hour internship in the areas of clinical and community nutrition and management. A registered dietician must also pass a national credentialing exam, and receive annual continuing education.

For further information on locating a registered dietician in your area who can provide professional nutrition consultation, or to get more information on basic nutrition concerns, call the American Dietetic Association's toll-free hotline: 800-366-1655. The organization also offers several free brochures on a wide variety of nutrition topics.

SEVEN

Tips for Tolerating
Lactose Intolerance

ERIN REFUSES TO LET LACTOSE INTOLERANCE GOVERN her life.

"When my doctor announced that my hydrogen breath test had come back positive, I swore right then that I wouldn't let the condition control my lifestyle," the 34-year-old dance instructor notes. "I didn't want to be one of those people whose very existence revolves around their medical disorder. Life has too much to offer to spend it fretting needlessly."

Erin talked with her doctor at length about how best to deal with the condition. He suggested she conduct a self-test to determine how much lactose she could handle before the onset of symptoms, and recommended that she keep lactase pills in her purse to cover those situations, such as parties and dining out, in which lactose levels were unknown.

"The best advice my doctor gave me, however, was not to worry about being lactose intolerant," Erin adds.

"He told me that millions of people have the condition, and that it would be fairly easy to deal with as long as I was careful and observant. And he was right. I watch my diet and work hard to keep my lactose intake to a minimum when I cook at home. As for parties and eating out, well, that's what lactase pills are for. Rather than having to beg off, they allow me to dive right in without having to worry about gas and bloating.

"To me, having lactose intolerance is like having bad eyesight. You may not be able to cure it, but you can adapt. For example, I've developed a dietary regimen at home that allows me to enjoy small amounts of my favorite dairy foods while maintaining proper nutrition with healthful nondairy alternatives. For example, I prepare a lot of Chinese, Thai, and Korean dishes because they are rich in vegetables, fish, and poultry and require very little milk or other dairy products. They're filling, nourishing, and my husband—who is not lactose intolerant—likes the wide variety they offer."

Erin refuses to dwell on the fact that she is lactose intolerant. To do so, she says, would mean that the condition has bested her. "I'm constantly aware of it," she states, "but I don't let it ruin my day. I know a lot of people whose lives are consumed by the fact that they are lactose intolerant. I don't want to be like that. Most of my friends aren't even aware that I have the condition. I eat just as well as they do when we go out, but my meals just happen to be lower in lactose than theirs—or I'll quietly take a few enzyme tablets to make digestion easier.

"Coping with lactose intolerance takes patience and perseverance, but it can be done. The most important thing to remember is that it's not the end of the world—although it may seem that way in the beginning. Most people with the condition can still enjoy a fair amount of dairy products, and there are several effective dietary aids on the market for those times when lactose levels become intolerable. As long as you're careful, the condition should have little impact on your health and happiness. I'm living proof of that!''

Erin is just one of millions of people who have learned to live comfortably with lactose intolerance. In this chapter, we'll offer easy and effective tips for tolerating lactose intolerance, with a special emphasis on foods that contain hidden lactose, words to look out for when grocery shopping, and how to take care of yourself when dining out or traveling.

Q: I was recently diagnosed with lactose intolerance, and the news sent me reeling. My doctor warned me to be cautious about the foods I eat, but she left me wondering: Do I have to give up all dairy products?

A: Definitely not. Yours is one of the most common concerns among people newly diagnosed with lactose intolerance. The good news is that people with all but the severest cases of lactose intolerance can still enjoy most dairy products—just not as much of them as they may be used to. As noted in Chapter One, lactose intolerance is not an all-or-nothing condition. The degree of intolerance varies widely among individuals with the problem, and very, very few are so intolerant that they can't eat any dairy at all. A lactose-free test, as discussed in Chapter Three, can help you determine exactly how much dairy you can you consume before the onset of symptoms.

And if you haven't already discovered the benefits of lactase pills, now's the time to do so. They come in several easy-to-use forms, and are usually quite effective in making the digestion of lactose easier. As long as you take a sufficient number of pills during your meal (you may have to experiment to find the number of pills that is right for you), you should be able to eat as much dairy as you want.

Q: Can you offer some additional tips on making the consumption of dairy products easier for people with lactose intolerance? I love dairy foods, but too much makes me sick. How can I hedge my bet against the onset of symptoms?

A: Eating below your lactose tolerance level or taking lactase pills with your meals is the best ways to prevent the onset of symptoms, but there are other helpful strategies as well. It should be noted, however, that lactase pills may work better for some people than for others. If you are extremely lactose intolerant (meaning that even tiny amounts of lactose induce symptoms), you may not find the pills quite as effective. Here are a few additional tips for making the consumption of dairy products easier:

- Consume milk or other dairy products with food, rather than by themselves. Nondairy foods can help buffer your system against the effects of lactose.
- If you absolutely must have dairy, consider yogurt with active cultures. Most yogurt is more easily tolerated by people with lactose intolerance.
- If you like cheese, select hard and/or aged varieties. They usually contain far lower levels of lactose than soft or processed cheeses.
- Whenever possible, substitute a lactose-reduced dairy product for one that is high in lactose.

Lactose-reduced products are labeled very clearly as such on their packaging.

Q: Can I build up a tolerance for lactose by eating a lot of it?

A: Possibly. Some research suggests that a regular diet of lactose-containing foods, specifically dairy products such as milk and cheese, may help create a shift in the type of bacteria in your colon, replacing those that create symptoms with those that don't.

The concept is based on the fact that a wide variety of bacteria exist in your colon. Some prefer an acidic environment, while others do not. Those that prefer a highly acidic environment include lactic acid bacteria such as *Lactobacillus* and *Streptococcus*, the same bacteria used in the manufacture of fermented-milk products like yogurt. They produce a lot of lactase but very little gas. Some researchers speculate that a daily dose of lactose can increase the population of these beneficial bacteria while reducing the population of those that cause problems, thus increasing your tolerance to lactose. At least, that's the theory.

The clinical research on this issue is mixed at best. However, a handful of studies have shown that it can work, at least in some people. In one study published in the journal *Gastroenterology*, 10 test subjects with lactose intolerance drank milk several times a day in an attempt to increase their total consumption. All experienced at least mild symptoms at the beginning of the experiment, but within weeks the majority could drink up to a quart of milk a day without an increase in digestive problems. Other studies noticed similar results.

Let me reiterate: Boosting lactose tolerance via the

regular consumption of lactose-containing foods doesn't work for everyone. The majority of people with lactose intolerance will not be able to develop increased tolerance, and will only torture themselves with aggravating symptoms if they try. Indeed, even people who succeed in increasing their tolerance to lactose through the regular consumption of milk report difficult symptoms during the first week or two.

Whether to attempt a tolerance boost is entirely up to you. It's possible that you may succeed, and that would certainly be a good thing. But it's more likely that you won't—especially if you are extremely lactose intolerant—and will endure needless symptoms. Before taking on such a challenge, it would be wise to discuss the issue with your doctor and get his input. As noted, there are easier ways to boost consumption of dairy products without increasing symptoms, such as consuming dairy with other foods and taking lactase pills with your meals. For most people with lactose intolerance, this is probably the wisest course of action.

Q: Could you provide a chart of the lactose content of common dairy foods? Such information would be helpful in determining how much of each can be safely consumed.
A: The lactose content of various foods can vary slightly from product to product and from manufacturer to manufacturer, but the following should give you an accurate average.

Content of Lactose Foods

Milk and Yogurt

Buttermilk (1 cup)	9–11 grams
Chocolate milk (1 cup)	10–12 grams
Eggnog (1 cup)	14 grams
Evaporated milk (undiluted) (1 cup)	20 grams
Goat milk (1 cup)	9.4 grams
Low-fat milk (1 cup)	9–13 grams
Low-sodium milk (1 cup)	9 grams
Nonfat dry milk powder (1 cup)	48 grams
Skim milk, fortified (1 cup)	12–14 grams
Sweetened condensed milk (1 cup)	35 grams
Whole milk (1 cup)	11 grams
Yogurt (1 cup)	11–15 grams

Cream

Cream cheese (1 ounce)	.6 gram
Half and half (½ cup)	5 grams
Heavy whipping cream (½ cup)	3 grams
Sour cream (½ cup)	3.2 grams

Spreads

Butter (1 tsp)	0.06 gram
Margarine (with milk solids) (1 tsp)	.9 grams

Cheese

Aged cheese (1 ounce)	.1–.8 gram
American cheese (1 ounce)	2.4 grams
Cheddar cheese (1 ounce)	.6 gram
Dry-curd cottage cheese (½ cup)	.8 gram
Low-fat cottage cheese (½ cup)	3.6 grams
Swiss cheese (1 ounce)	.5 gram

Desserts

Fudge Bar	4.9 grams
Ice cream (½ cup)	5–7 grams
Ice-cream sandwich	2.4 grams
Ice milk (½ cup)	6–7.5 grams
Ices (½ cup)	0 grams
Milk chocolate (3 ounces)	8.1 grams
Orange Creme Bar	3.1 grams
Sherbet (½ cup)	2 grams

Q: I seem to tolerate chocolate milk a little better than regular milk. Why is this?

A: Many people with lactose intolerance find that they can tolerate chocolate milk a little more easily than regular milk—good news if you're a real milk lover and want to keep it a part of your diet. However, the reason behind this increased tolerance is a subject of debate. Some nutrition experts speculate that the addition of cocoa solids to milk reduces the lactose level by a small but significant percentage. Others theorize that cocoa solids move lactose through the intestines at a slower rate, so lactase has more time to act upon it.

Q: Why do aged or hard cheeses have a lower lactose level than soft cheeses? They're both made from milk, so the discrepancy doesn't make sense. After all, cheese is cheese.

A: Cheese may be cheese, but how it's made can result in a big difference in lactose levels. Most cheeses are made by adding a special enzyme to coagulate (to change from a fluid to a solid state) the milk protein called casein. This separates the milk into two parts—curds (the solid part) and whey (the liquid part). The majority of cheeses consumed in the United States are made from the curd.

Soft cheeses are made by halting the cheese-making process right after the curd separates. Most soft cheeses are very high in lactose because a lot of whey is incorporated into the curds. Harder cheeses are made by removing more whey from the curds (the more whey that is discarded, the lower the lactose level of a particular cheese). The cheeses are then aged using molds or bacteria, which give a specific cheese its unique flavor. As a rule of thumb, the longer a cheese ages, or ripens, the more intense, or sharp, its flavor—and the lower its lactose level.

Q: Is it true that yogurt is actually good for lactose intolerance? If so, what makes it more tolerable than other dairy products?

A: Yogurt, which is made by fermenting milk with special bacterial cultures, is one of the oldest dairy products known to man—and one of the best tolerated among individuals with lactose intolerance. It was first made in the Middle East nearly 5,000 years ago as a way of keeping milk from spoiling (yogurt remained edible for weeks despite the lack of refrigeration), and it quickly became a nutritional mainstay of that region. Yogurt in its varied forms is mentioned in numerous ancient texts, including the Old Testament of the Bible— Abraham offered sweet and sour milk (yogurt) to visiting angels.

Yogurt in its traditional form tends to be on the sour side because of a by-product known as lactic acid, so it wasn't particularly popular in the United States until the 1940s when the Dannon Corporation wisely added fruit as a sweetener. But even then, sales didn't exactly go through the roof. In fact, yogurt didn't really catch on in the United States until the 1970s, when everyone started clamoring for health foods. Low-fat yogurts also boosted sales. Today, yogurt is one of the most popular dairy products available and can be found in a wide variety of forms and flavors.

Yogurt is made by first concentrating whole, low-fat, or nonfat milk with additional milk solids to thicken the mixture during the manufacturing process. This makes the base formula even higher in lactose than plain milk, but people with lactose intolerance needn't worry—everything works out okay in the end. The milk is then pasteurized (heated) to kill unwanted bacteria, and various types of beneficial bacteria are added for fermentation. The most common types of bacteria used in the manufacture of yogurt are *Lactobacillus bulgaricus* and *Streptococcus thermophilus,* though sometimes *Lactobacillus acidophilus* is also used. The bacteria ferment the milk and harden the casein protein into creamy curds. They also produce lactase, which breaks down much of the lactose that came with the additional milk solids. Once the yogurt has achieved a specific tartness and texture, it is refrigerated to halt the fermentation process. This also prevents the bacteria from producing any more lactase.

So why is yogurt better tolerated than many other dairy products? Because the bacteria-produced lactase is delivered to the intestines when you eat it, allowing for easier digestion. Most other enzymes are destroyed by stomach acid, but for reasons still unexplained, yogurt protects the lactase just enough to allow it to make its way to the duodenum (the first part of the small intestine), where the breakdown of lactose occurs. The lactase levels of most yogurt products are high enough that almost all of the lactose can be digested, and the amount that eventually makes its way to the colon is usually so small that it produces few if any symptoms in all but the most extreme cases of lactose intolerance.

Several clinical studies have confirmed the digestibility of yogurt among people with lactose intolerance. In one study, researchers fed 18 grams of lactose in yogurt, milk, and water to people with lactose intolerance and found that only one-third the level of breath hydrogen was recorded after consuming yogurt compared to the consumption of lactose in water or milk. And in a second study, breath hydrogen levels, blood glucose levels, insulin, and free fatty acid levels were measured after lactose, milk, sweet acidophilus milk, yogurt, or heat-treated fermented milk were fed to volunteers with and without lactose intolerance. All with lactose intolerance reported no symptoms when they consumed yogurt.

Q: Can eating yogurt with other dairy products result in fewer symptoms? In other words, can the lactase in yogurt help digest the lactose in other foods?
A: Usually not. The amount of lactase in yogurt is usually sufficient to digest only that amount of lactose and no more. So eating yogurt while drinking a large glass of milk will probably still result in symptoms because a good amount of lactose will likely reach the colon.

Q: Are all yogurts equal regarding lactase-producing bacteria? Is there anything we should look for on the label to make sure we're getting the greatest benefit?

A: All yogurts are not created equal. Most say "made with active cultures," but that really doesn't mean much because many yogurt products are reheated for a longer shelf life following the fermentation process, killing the beneficial bacteria.

To make sure you're getting the best kind of yogurt for people with lactose intolerance, look for a statement regarding live, active cultures on the label. "Made with" and "contains" are two different things. All yogurt is made with live cultures, but only those still containing live, active cultures can say so on the label. It's also a good sign if a product contains the National Yogurt Association's Live and Active Cultures logo. Avoid products that say "heat-treated after culturing" because they do not contain active cultures. As for the inclusion of fruit, flavorings, and other additives, they should have no effect on live cultures.

Q: Do frozen and soft-serve yogurt desserts also contain live, active cultures? Are they as well tolerated by people with lactose intolerance as plain, refrigerated yogurt?

A: Frozen yogurt can make a great dessert or snack treat, but as with refrigerated yogurt, you have to read the label carefully to determine whether it contains active cultures (again, the National Yogurt Association's Live and Active Cultures logo makes a good guide). Nutrition experts note that even if frozen yogurt does contain active cultures, there's no guarantee that the cultures will work as well in your digestive tract.

The problem is that many frozen yogurt products undergo a second pasteurization to extend shelf life prior to freezing. This kills the beneficial bacteria. Some manufacturers try to make things better by adding starter cultures immediately before freezing, but there is evidence that this doesn't really give the cultures sufficient time to produce lactase. A study reported in the journal *Dairy Foods* concluded that refrigerated yogurts have the highest amounts of active cultures, with hard-pack frozen yogurt second and soft-serve yogurt a distant third. Bottom line: Fresh refrigerated yogurt may have up to 1,000 times the amount of active cultures as frozen yogurt products. People with lactose intolerance may have to do a little experimentation to determine which frozen yogurt products are best tolerated by their digestive system.

Q: I have severe lactose intolerance, and my doctor warned me about "hidden lactose" in commercial food products. How common is this problem, and what kinds of foods are most likely to contain hidden lactose?

A: You'd be surprised at the number of foods in your pantry that probably contain milk, milk by-products, or straight lactose. In many, the amount is so small as to be inconsequential. But in others, it can be enough to potentially trigger symptoms in people with lactose intolerance. That's why it's often helpful to take lactase pills with every meal, regardless of what's on the menu.

A small sampling of foods that you wouldn't think contain lactose but do:

- **Bread and other baked goods.** The inclusion of lactose in a particular bread or other baked good varies dramatically from manufacturer to manufacturer, and from product to product; some do, some don't. As general rule, however, white breads, hamburger rolls, and hot dog rolls are usually made with at least a small amount of milk, but crusty breads and rolls such as French bread, Italian bread, pumpernickel, and rye are lactose free (so are soft versions of traditionally crusty breads). Make sure you carefully read the list of ingredients before making your purchase. Some companies make milk-free white bread, but it can be difficult to find in many parts of the country.

- **Processed breakfast cereals.** Many popular breakfast cereals contain milk products, including nonfat milk, whey, and nonfat dry milk. Again, read the list of ingredients to find out which do and which don't. Relatively speaking, however, this is a minor issue. The amount of milk products found in most breakfast cereals tends to be small and should pose little problem for people with mild to moderate lactose intolerance. Traditional cream of wheat and cream of rice, despite their names, contain no dairy products—though some flavored instant versions do.

- **Instant potatoes, soups, and breakfast drinks.** A wide variety of "instant" foods are made with milk products, and some of them contain fairly high amounts, so be careful. Many canned soups—especially the "cream of" varieties and most seafood chowders—are also made with milk, and may contain a potentially high level of lactose. The one exception is Manhattan clam chowder, which has a tomato base and is lactose-free. Clear soups such as broth and bouillon also contain no lactose.

- **Lunch meats (other than kosher).** Nonfat dry milk is a common filler ingredient in many hot dogs and processed lunch meats, such as salami, so read the label carefully. The best way to make sure your lunch meats are lactose-free is to buy the kosher varieties—they are guaranteed not to contain any milk products.

- **Salad dressings.** The worst offenders are buttermilk, ranch, or caesar-style dressings—almost all of them contain milk or cheese as an integral ingredient. People with lactose intolerance are encouraged to stick to oil-and-vinegar or mayonnaise-based dressings, which are almost entirely lactose-free—even if they are the "creamy" variety.

- **Candies and other snacks.** A surprisingly high number of candies contain milk, including true butterscotch. Clear, hard candies such as sour balls and lollipops are a safe alternative for people with lactose intolerance. So is licorice. As for snacks, pretzels and regular potato chips are usually lactose-free, though potato chips and other snacks with dip flavorings added, such as sour cream and onion, ranch or nacho cheese, are made with milk products and should be avoided. Butter-flavored popcorn is usually made with vegetable oil and thus is safe for people with lactose intolerance.

- **Mixes for pancakes, biscuits, cakes, and cookies.** One might assume that mixes for baked goods would be packed with dairy products, but a surprisingly high number are actually lactose-free—though you should still read the ingredients list just to make sure. Mixes containing milk chocolate or chocolate bits usually contain dairy products, but these are a small minority. People with lactose intolerance should also be wary of so-called flavored cake mixes; most contain at least a small amount of milk products.

- **Fruit juices, carbonated drinks, and other beverages.** Lactose and lactose-containing milk products are occasionally used as an ingredient in processed fruit juices and certain carbonated beverages. Read the list of ingredients to make sure you're buying a brand that is milk-free. So-called cream sodas are not made with milk and thus are safe for people with lactose intolerance. So are crème de menthe and crème de cacao. But if a product spells the word "cream" correctly, beware. It probably contains real cream.

- **Spices.** A small number of spices use lactose to prevent caking, but this is becoming increasingly less common. However, packaged spice mixes for use in chili or tacos often contain milk products, though dairy-free alternatives are also available. Cream of tartar, despite its name, contains no cream or other milk products.

- **Canned foods.** A wide variety of canned and jarred foods contain milk products. A few common examples include spaghetti sauce with cheese, canned pasta meals, chicken stews (especially those in a milk-based sauce) and ready-to-heat gravies. If you're in doubt, read the label.

As you can see, dairy products are a popular ingredient in many common food items. So is pure lactose because it makes a terrific thickener for soups, gravies, and sauces. Manufacturers prefer it to cornstarch and flour because it dissolves almost immediately; it doesn't cake, clump or add unwanted sweetness; and is relatively innocuous—unless you have lactose intolerance. Lactose is also used to make the production of certain foods easier and to improve texture and appearance of various products.

Q: What should people with lactose intolerance look for on food labels to determine if a product contains lactose?

A: There are a number of words and phrases that should give people with lactose intolerance reason to pause. The most common are whey, curds, milk by-products, dry milk solids, and nonfat dry milk powder. If any of these are listed on a food label, the item contains lactose and should be consumed with caution. Let's break these words down for a clearer understanding of what they are and how they can affect people with lactose intolerance.

- **Whey.** As noted earlier, whey is the liquid that's left over when solid curds form during the manufacture of cheese. Fresh liquid whey contains about 93 percent water, 5 percent lactose and 2 percent milk proteins and various nutrients. Whey is used in a tremendous number of food products, usually in a dry form that has a much higher level of lactose than liquid whey (removing the water from liquid whey leaves a very concentrated powder). In fact, the lactose content of whey is so high that most commercial lactose is derived from it.

  The U.S. Food and Drug Administration allows three forms of whey to be used in the manufacture of food: concentrated whey, reconstituted whey, and dried whey. There is rarely a distinction between them on food labels, however, because the FDA allows them all to be identified solely as "whey." In addition, very few food labels tell consumers exactly how much whey a particular product contains, which makes shopping a difficult task for people with lactose intolerance. As a rule of thumb, however, if you see the word *whey* on a label, expect a relatively high lactose level. And if it's one of the first three ingredients listed, expect a very high lactose level.

- **Curds.** The semisoft by-product that results from the coagulation of a milk protein known as casein (whey is the liquid by-product), curds are usually associated with various cheese products, such as cottage cheese and ricotta cheese. Curds are safer for people with lactose intolerance because they contain far less lactose than whey. However, curds are not lactose-free.

- **Milk solids.** This is an umbrella term for just about everything in milk except the water. It includes protein, fat, vitamins, minerals, and lactose (lactose is nutritionally referred to as a carbohydrate).

- **Milk fats.** Products made from milk fats, such as butter, tend to be very low in lactose and are generally better tolerated by people with lactose intolerance. Many foods are made with milk fat, which may also be known as butter fat or butter oil, and most pose few problems to people with lactose intolerance.

  Milk fat may be disguised on product labels as saturated fatty acids (which include myristic acid, palmitic acid, and stearic acid) or unsaturated fatty acids (which include oleic acid, linoleic acid, and linolenic acid). Again, all of these are low in lactose and relatively safe for people with lactose intolerance.

- **Milk proteins.** Although protein is a very small part of the nutritional makeup of milk, dietary experts say it is vital to proper nutrition. More than 75 percent of milk protein comes from casein (a milk protein), which is important in the manufacture of cheese. Casein tends to collect in the curds, so the protein content of many cheeses is higher than that of the milk from which it is made. Because casein is so high in protein, many manufacturers add it to their food products to boost protein levels on the nutrition label. It is also a common component of many nondairy products.

Casein by itself shouldn't affect most people with lactose intolerance. It may have a tiny amount of lactose attached to it during processing, but usually the level is so small as to be inconsequential. However, people who are allergic to cow's milk protein, as discussed in Chapter Three, should avoid all products known to have casein in them, including those labeled "nondairy." In extremely sensitive individuals, even a small amount of casein can trigger a severe and potentially life-threatening allergic reaction.

Additional milk proteins are derived from whey. Two types of whey-based proteins are most common: the lactalbumins and the lactoglobulins. Both can cause a reaction in people with milk-protein allergies, but rarely affect people with lactose intolerance. Stay away from products that contain whey-protein concentrate, however. It is high in lactose and could trigger symptoms in sensitive people.

Q: Almost every food label I read in the grocery store contains at least one of the dairy components listed above. How can I reduce my chances of buying

something that's going to trigger symptoms of lactose intolerance?

A: Shopping can be tricky for people with lactose intolerance. As you've noted, it seems that many foods on store shelves these days contains some component of milk. But you can make things easier by carefully reading the ingredients label. The reason: The placement of these items will give you a good indication of how much lactose a particular item contains. For example, if a dairy product is one of the first three ingredients on the list, it will probably contain a high level of lactose and should be avoided. According to nutrition experts, you should also be wary if:

- Dried whey or dried milk is one of the first five ingredients.
- A product contains dried whey or dried milk plus another dairy product, or three or more dairy products in any form.
- The food in question contains a high number of dairy ingredients and is something you're likely to pig out on. The more you eat, the more lactose you're going to be feeding your body—and the more symptoms you're likely to encounter. If your favorite foods are high-lactose items, consider dairy-free or lactose-reduced alternatives, or take lactase pills whenever you eat them.

Q: I noticed recently that a particular food item I purchased at my local grocery contains "lactic acid." Is this compound safe for people with lactose intolerance?

A: Absolutely. Lactic acid is a by-product of bacterial lactose fermentation in cultured milk products such as yogurt, and helps give such products their tart flavor. It's easy to understand your confusion—lactic acid sounds a lot like lactose—but lactic acid contains virtually no lactose, and thus is perfectly safe for people with lactose intolerance.

Q: I've noticed that the labels on a few products, such as certain cheeses, say they contain 0% lactose per serving. Does this mean they are lactose-free?

A: Not necessarily. A product may say that it contains 0% lactose and still contain the popular milk sugar, though usually in quantities so small as to be meaningless to most people with lactose intolerance. The label is technically correct because the Food and Drug Administration (FDA) regulations recognize that absolutes are difficult to achieve in the manufacture of food, so products labeled 0% this or that are still allowed to contain minuscule amounts of the ingredient in question. For all intents and purposes, however, the amount is 0%. However, a product cannot say that it is lactose-free unless it contains absolutely no lactose. There's a small but very important distinction between the two statements.

Q: Can an emphasis on kosher products help control the amount of lactose in my diet? A friend told me that many kosher foods contain no dairy products.

A: Your friend is right. Kosher foods can be a blessing for people with lactose intolerance because by Jewish dietary law, kosher foods cannot mix meat and dairy (though they can be one or the other). Neutral foods, meaning those that contain no meat or milk at all, are known as *pareve* or *parve* and are usually—but not always—marked as such on their packaging; it's up to the manufacturer. Pareve foods are completely lactose-free because they are completely milk-free. Examples include fish, eggs, fruits, and vegetables, as well as processed foods that contain no dairy or meat products. (Only fish that has both fins and scales is permitted and shellfish, such as lobsters, oysters, crabs, and shrimp, is not permitted.)

It's important to note the distinction between kosher and pareve foods. They aren't interchangeable. Pareve foods contain no meat or dairy, while kosher is a religious term with a specific religious meaning determined by specific religious criteria; it's not an ethnic way of cooking as many people believe.

One of the most important concepts in Jewish dietary law governs the selection, preparation, and slaughter of animals. Only four-footed animals that both chew their cud and have cloven feet may be eaten. This includes cattle, sheep, goats, and deer, but not pigs because pigs don't chew their cud. Fowl such as chicken, turkey, goose, and duck are allowed, but birds of prey are not. All animals must be free of any physical blemishes in order to be certified kosher.

Animals must be slaughtered according to specific religious laws. Animals that died of natural causes or were not slaughtered according to the prescribed Jewish ritual may not be labeled kosher. Jewish dietary law also forbids blood as food, so slaughtered animals and fowl must have all blood removed via soaking and salting, then be washed under cold running water, a process that is known as "koshering." Many kosher meat markets and delis sell fresh and frozen prekoshered meat and fowl.

Another concept integral to the rules of *kashrut* (the Jewish dietary laws)—and one that greatly benefits individuals with lactose intolerance—is the separation of meat and dairy products. Meat and meat products may not be eaten with dairy products in the same meal, and in many strictly kosher households, if meat is eaten first, one to six hours must elapse before dairy products can be consumed. In many Jewish households, the dairy meal (known as *milchig*) is the midday meal, and the meat meal (known as *fleischig*) is the evening meal. Pareve foods, because they contain neither meat nor milk, can be consumed with both.

Because of this rule of separation, kosher processed meats are guaranteed not to contain milk products and can be safely consumed by people with lactose intolerance. Such products can be found in the meat section of most supermarkets, as well as in kosher delis and butcher shops. In fact, many doctors encourage their patients with lactose intolerance to do as much of their shopping as possible at kosher delis and stores because they know that all processed meat products are free of dairy.

If you don't have a kosher store in your neighborhood, don't worry—many food manufacturers prepare their products according to kosher food laws. However, there is no single overseeing body, so products may contain any one of a number of identifying symbols, known as *hechshers*. The "U" in a circle, which is the stamp of the Union of Orthodox Jewish Congregations, is one of the best recognized and most respected symbols for kosher food. A "U" in a circle followed by a "D" has two meanings: that the food is kosher and contains dairy products, or that it is kosher and contains no milk products, but was manufactured with the same machinery used to make dairy products. You may also find some foods marked with a "U,P" symbol. This "P" does not stand for "pareve" but means that the food is kosher for Passover, a holiday that has additional dietary laws.

Q: I love dairy products but my lactose intolerance prevents me from consuming large amounts. I've tried lactase pills, but often forget to take them until it's too late. My doctor told me that there is a wide variety of so-called alternative dairy products for people like me. Could you discuss some of the most common?

A: Sure. The truth is, most of the manufacturers of dairy products are well aware of the huge number of people who cannot tolerate lactose and are trying to tap into that potentially lucrative market with various lactose-reduced or nondairy alternatives. Lactose-reduced milk is one of the larger areas, but there is also substitute butter, ice cream, and more. Following is a brief look at what's currently available:

• **Milks.** We've already discussed reduced-lactose milks—the kind that have lactase added during processing to make them easier to digest. Several companies manufacture reduced-lactose milk and they're fairy easy to find in grocery dairy departments. But there are also nondairy milk alternatives that can be beneficial to people with lactose intolerance. Some of the most common are nondairy creamers and whipped toppings. Nondairy creamers can be used instead of milk to flavor coffee and other beverages and can sometimes be used in place of milk on foods like dry cereal. However, while many such products have nutrients added, they are usually not as nutritious as regular milk and it is unwise to rely on them for essential nutrients such as calcium. In addition, many nondairy creamers are a source of saturated fats. The most healthful are those that contain a vegetable oil, such as cottonseed or soybean oil, as the fat source. The same goes for nondairy whipped toppings.

Many alternative milk products contain the milk protein casein but are relatively low in lactose and thus okay for people with lactose intolerance (however, just to be on the safe side, it's always wise to read the ingredients label for telltale words that could suggest a higher than desirable lactose level). The latest trend in the area of alternative milk products is flavored nondairy creamers. All of these products use milk protein, and some use whey protein as well as casein, which makes them risky for people with milk protein allergies. However, they are an effective milk substitute for those with only lactose intolerance.

- **Butters.** Because natural butters are high in fat, they tend to be very low in lactose (the range averages from 0.8 to 1.0 percent). As a result, most people with lactose intolerance can consume moderate amounts of butter without having to worry about symptoms. But for those who don't want to risk even that, there's margarine, which is usually made with more vegetable oil than milk and thus is a nice substitute for people with extreme lactose intolerance. Margarine has had a rough history—in the early days, dairy producers fought hard to keep it off the market—but today it can be found in a variety of types and forms, including sticks, tubs, and even squeeze bottles. Most margarines still contain at least a little dairy for flavor, but the lactose content is extremely small, ranging from 0.0 to 1.0 percent. For those looking for butters that are completely dairy-free, many health food stores carry alternative butters made with canola oil or soybean oil.

- **Cheeses.** Cheese doesn't pose quite the same problem as other dairy products for people with lactose intolerance. Aged cheese, in particular, tends to be very low in lactose and easily tolerated by people with the condition. However, for those who don't want to take any chances, there are several brands of cheese that are made with soy and other nondairy ingredients that look and taste almost like the real thing (though some of them don't cook quite as well as regular cheese). Most alternative cheeses contain at least a small amount of the milk protein casein, but for all intents and purposes, they are lactose-free.

- **Ice cream.** As noted earlier, true reduced-lactose ice cream can be difficult to find. Many manufacturers have tried their hand at it, but consumer interest has always been tepid, possibly because reduced-lactose ice cream just doesn't taste the same as regular ice cream. However, there are a lot of nondairy frozen desserts on the market that are manufactured with dairy substitutes such as tofu, which is made from curdled soybean milk. (Don't let the word *milk* fool you, though. It's a vegetable derivative that contains no lactose.) The first tofu frozen dessert was introduced in 1976, but the idea didn't really catch on until the introduction of Tofutti Brand Non-Dairy Frozen Dessert in 1982. The public loved the stuff—especially people with lactose intolerance—and pretty soon the marketplace was flooded with competitors. When the dust settled, one of the few remaining brands still in su-

permarkets was the one that started it all: Tofutti.
Frozen tofu products remain popular in health food
stores, but frozen yogurt—another tasty, low-
lactose ice cream substitute—has pretty much taken
over the market in larger grocery stores and supermarkets.

- **Yogurt.** Because it has active bacterial cultures, yogurt is one dairy product that is usually well tolerated by people with lactose intolerance. However,
many health food stores and even some groceries
and supermarkets carry nondairy yogurt made with
soy or a combination of soy and rice. Most are
made with the same healthful bacterial cultures,
which makes them doubly good for people with lactose intolerance.

**Q: Is soy milk a nutritious substitute for cow's milk?
Is it good for people with lactose intolerance?**
A: Soy milk is commonly used as a substitute for cow's
milk in many Asian countries, and its popularity continues to rise in the United States as more and more people
look for healthful food alternatives. It's good for people
with lactose intolerance because it contains no lactose.

Soy milk is easy to manufacture. Soybeans (which are
legumes) are presoaked, then ground with water into a
puree. The paste is mixed with hot water, cooked for a
few minutes, then strained and pressed. The resulting
white elixir is known as soy milk.

Soy milk is extremely nutritious, but not quite as nutritious as regular milk. It is very low in fat, cholesterol-
free, and rich in protein. Many commercial brands of
soy milk are also fortified with essential nutrients found
in regular milk, including potassium, calcium, vitamin
A and vitamin C. In addition, soy milk is the base for a

nutritious, dairy-free infant formula. However, regular soy milk by itself should not be given to babies; while it does contain important nutrients, malnutrition can result if soy milk is an infant's only food source.

Soy milk can often be used in place of regular milk in many recipes. However, you should always use unflavored soy milk so that the recipe doesn't end up tasting like the flavoring used in the soy milk. Many Asian dishes rely on soy milk instead of regular milk because lactose intolerance is such a big problem among Asian populations.

Certain fruits and nuts also provide effective milk substitutes, although most are unfamiliar to the majority of Americans. Probably the best known is coconut milk which, like soy, is still commonly used in Asian cuisine. Native Americans derived a milklike liquid from hickory, pecans, and other nuts for use in cooking, and in Europe, walnuts and almonds were pulverized and soaked in water to produce a milk substitute that had a variety of uses. Of course, these vegetable-produced milks are seldom seen anymore because of the dominance of cow and other animal milk.

Q: I told my pharmacist that I was lactose intolerant, and she warned me that a lot of prescription and over-the-counter medications contain lactose. Is this true?

A: Yes. Lactose makes a great base or filler for medications sold in capsule and pill form because it is flavorless, dissolves easily, and, most importantly, doesn't cake or clump. It's also a very safe and innocuous substance—unless you have lactose intolerance. According to the National Institute of Diabetes and Digestive and Kidney Diseases (NIDDK), more than 20 percent of prescription medications and nearly 6 percent of over-the-counter medications contain lactose as a base.

This may sound problematic, but the fact of the matter is that the amount of lactose used in the manufacture of prescription and over-the-counter medications is minuscule and of little concern to the majority of people with lactose intolerance. Most people will never feel a thing, although individuals with a severe form of the condition may experience symptoms, especially if they take several pills a day (a common problem among the elderly). People with galactosemia and related disorders are also at high risk because they must maintain a completely lactose-free diet. (See Chapter Three for more information on this disease.)

Most medications, especially those sold over the counter, list all of their inactive ingredients, so it's wise to read the label before making a purchase. If you are taking prescription medications, make sure both your doctor and your pharmacist are aware of your lactose intolerance so that they can take steps to ensure that the medications you receive are as lactose-free as possible. In most cases, alternative forms are available for the asking. If your doctor is reluctant to switch medications because he is comfortable with one brand and that's what he's always prescribed, get a second opinion. You have the right to lactose-free medications if you want and need them. But be aware that refusing all of the medications your doctor recommends simply because they may contain a little lactose could compromise your doctor's ability to treat you effectively.

Hundreds of medications contain lactose as an inactive ingredient. Some of the most common include:

Anaprox (arthritis medication)
Ativan (antianxiety agent)

Benadryl (over-the-counter antihistamine)

Bentyl (antispasmodic medication used in the treatment of gastrointestinal problems)

Buspar (antianxiety agent)

Cardene SR (calcium channel blocker used in the treatment of certain heart conditions)

Catapres (cardiovascular agent)

Claritin (antihistamine)

Compazine (antinausea medication)

Cylert (central nervous system stimulant)

Darvon-N (narcotic painkiller)

Dilantin (antiseizure medication)

Ducolax (over-the-counter laxative)

Elavil (antidepressant)

Eldepryl (used in the treatment of Parkinson's disease)

Feldene (arthritis medication)

Flexeril (muscle relaxant)

Hydrocortone (anti-inflammatory agent)

Imodium (over-the-counter diarrhea medication)

Inderal (beta blocker used in the treatment of certain heart conditions)

Klonopin (antiseizure medication)

Lasix (heart medication/diuretic)

Levothroid (synthetic thyroid medication)

Librium (antianxiety agent)

Lodine (arthritis medication)

Lopressor (beta blocker used in the treatment of certain heart conditions)

Moban (antipsychotic medication)

Nembutol Sodium (sedative)

Nitrostat (vasodilator used in the treatment of certain heart conditions)

Ortho-Cept (oral contraceptive)

Ortho-Cyclen (oral contraceptive)

Ortho-Novum (oral contraceptive)

Parnate (antidepressant)

Phenergan (antihistamine, motion sickness medication)

Phenobarbital (sedative, antiseizure medication)

Premarin (estrogen supplement)

Proscar (used in the treatment of prostatic hypertrophy)

Provera (progestogen supplement)

Restoril (sedative)

Rheumatrex (arthritis medication)

Serax (antianxiety medication)

Synthroid (synthetic thyroid medication)

Tavist (antihistamine)

Thorazine (antipsychotic medication, also used to ease nausea)

Triphasil (oral contraceptive)

Vasotec (vasodilator used in the treatment of certain heart conditions)

Wigraine (migraine headache medication)

Xanax (antianxiety medication)

Zocor (cholesterol-lowering medication)

Zovirax (antiviral medication used in the treatment of herpes)

(Note: Many of the medications listed above, as well as those not listed, are available in variations that do not contain lactose, usually injectibles or drops. Ask your doctor about nonlactose-containing alternatives.)

Q: I enjoy eating out with family and friends, but my lactose intolerance presents a problem. What advice can you offer to make dining out easier for people with my condition?

A: Whether it's in a fast-food restaurant or a four-star restaurant, dining out can be a digestive minefield for people with lactose intolerance because, with rare exceptions, you seldom know exactly what goes into the foods you're eating. Many processed foods contain lactose, and it's not uncommon for chefs to add milk, cream, or other dairy products to their dishes, especially sauces.

The most obvious answer is to take lactase pills throughout your meal on the assumption that it's packed with lactose. That way, you can eat pretty much whatever you want without having to worry about the after-effects. It may also help to mention to your waiter that you're lactose intolerant (you may have to explain what that means) and ask him to recommend dishes that contain little if any dairy.

If neither of these suggestions is an option, keep your selections simple—broiled chicken, meat, or seafood; steamed vegetables; salad with oil-and-vinegar dressing; plain coffee or iced tea; and sorbet for dessert. A menu like this should contain little to no lactose, especially if you avoid gravies and sauces, which more often than not are prepared with milk, cream, or cheese.

A similar approach can also help you avoid hidden lactose when eating in fast-food restaurants. If available, get grilled or broiled chicken, a baked potato (with just a dab of butter for flavor) and/or the salad bar (stick with oil-and-vinegar dressing—it's your safest bet). Regardless of what type of fast-food place you're in—hamburgers, Mexican, barbecue—study the menu carefully before ordering.

In addition, the type of restaurant you select when dining out can be helpful in avoiding lactose. We've mentioned the benefits of Asian cuisine often in this book, and for good reason—most Japanese, Chinese, Thai, and Korean dishes contain little if any dairy, though you should be careful about dessert. Kosher restaurants and delis (but obviously not kosher dairy restaurants) are also fairly safe, as are vegetarian restaurants. But stay away from Italian and French restaurants, which commonly incorporate cheese, milk, and cream into their traditional fare.

Q: I travel frequently as part of my job, and spend several weeks a year doing business in foreign countries. I also have fairly severe lactose intolerance. Any tips to make my travels a little easier on my digestive tract?

A: Make sure you pack plenty of lactase supplements; in times of dining uncertainty, they can be a real lifesaver. Pills or capsules that can be opened are recommended because they travel well and don't require refrigeration. Stock up on your favorite brand, but don't fret if you run out because lactase supplements and lactose-reduced dairy products usually can be found in the larger cities of most industrialized nations.

Some areas of the world, of course, present more of a problem than others to people with lactose intolerance. Most European cuisine can be counted on to contain a fair amount of dairy products. South and Central American cuisine may also contain some lactose, but traditionally is more meat, vegetable, and legume oriented. African and Asian cuisine typically contain very little dairy, but there are always exceptions so ask if you're uncertain. And Australian cuisine tends to be very much like American food, which means a relatively high lactose content.

If you don't speak the language of the country you're

visiting, bring a phrase book and learn how to describe your condition, ask about ingredients, and request non-dairy alternatives if necessary. Most restaurants will be happy to oblige.

EIGHT

Lactose Intolerance and
Special Populations

JENNIFER AND HER HUSBAND, TED, HAD TALKED FOR
more than a year about starting a family. They discussed
various considerations, such as whether they should look
for a larger house and the impact a child would have on
their lifestyle, and decided that the time was right. Two
months later, Jennifer received the good news from her
gynecologist—she was pregnant.

"I was ecstatic, but one thing started to worry me that
I hadn't considered before," recalls the 28-year-old mas-
sage therapist. "I have fairly severe lactose intolerance,
and I was concerned that the condition would impact on
my pregnancy or somehow affect my unborn baby."

Jennifer discussed her fears with her obstetrician during her initial examination, and breathed a heavy sigh
of relief when her doctor told her she had nothing to
worry about.

"We discussed my lactose intolerance, and I explained how I keep the condition under control by lim-

iting my consumption of dairy products and taking lactase pills with meals. My doctor reassured me that the condition itself should have no effect on my baby's growth and development, but she did suggest I reevaluate my diet to make sure that I got all of the calcium and other nutrients my baby and I would need for a healthy pregnancy. She gave me a list of calcium-rich nondairy foods, and she also encouraged me to take prenatal vitamins.''

Jennifer's mother, Patricia, is also lactose intolerant. Like Jennifer, she keeps symptoms to a minimum by avoiding lactose-containing foods and taking lactase pills with her meals. Patricia's doctor, like Jennifer's, also expressed concern that her condition was inhibiting her consumption of essential nutrients and threatening her future health.

"The smallest amounts of lactose make me extremely sick, so I've spent most of my life trying to avoid dairy products,'' says the 49-year-old part-time police dispatcher. "Then I compounded the problem by filling the rest of my diet with fried foods, red meat, and very few vegetables. This meant I wasn't getting anywhere near enough calcium and other nutrients, a situation that placed me at high risk of developing osteoporosis. I'm rapidly approaching menopause, so on my doctor's advice I'm taking calcium supplements every day, packing my meals with more nutritious foods, and working out at a gym four days a week. If I'm lucky, I shouldn't have too many problems when menopause arrives.''

Jennifer and Patricia were lucky—they discovered the potential impact of lactose intolerance on their unique situations (pregnancy and impending menopause) before it was too late. In this chapter, we'll discuss at length how lactose intolerance can affect special populations, with an emphasis on pregnant women, children, and the elderly.

Q: I was diagnosed with lactose intolerance five years ago, and manage my condition well through dietary control and the use of lactase supplements. My husband and I have been trying to start a family for months, and I just found out that I'm five weeks pregnant. Now I'm worried that my lactose intolerance could somehow affect my unborn baby. Should I be concerned?

A: No. Lactose intolerance is a common medical condition that makes the digestion of lactose difficult. It affects only the digestive system and has no effect at all on a woman's reproductive organs, so your condition should have no impact on the growth and development of your unborn baby. Lactose intolerance is not a disease, so it cannot be spread from mother to child. Your baby may eventually grow up to be lactose intolerant, but that's because of genetics, not anything you did or didn't do during your pregnancy.

Q: Could you please discuss the effects of lactose intolerance on nutrition during pregnancy? It's my understanding that lactose intolerant women should take special dietary precautions during pregnancy to make sure that they and their unborn babies get plenty of essential nutrients.

A: You're absolutely right—proper nutrition is vital during all stages of pregnancy, and women with lactose intolerance must take extra steps to ensure that they are eating well.

One of the biggest problems facing women with lactose intolerance is the avoidance of dairy products. Most people with the condition can consume at least small amounts of dairy, but it's not uncommon for sufferers to avoid all dairy as an easy way of preventing symptoms. However, milk and other dairy products are a primary source of many nutrients that are important to both a pregnant woman and her unborn child, such as calcium, vitamin D, and protein, and women who avoid dairy must look elsewhere for those nutrients. Poor nutrition can sometimes lead to miscarriage, and in addition, unborn babies deprived of essential nutrients may not develop properly and could experience health problems that will last them the rest of their lives.

We discussed the importance of nutrition during pregnancy in Chapter Six, but let's briefly review the most essential nutrients traditionally derived from milk and the nondairy sources in which they can be found.

- **Calcium.** Necessary for the growth and development of a baby's bones and teeth. Women need 1,200 milligrams a day during pregnancy and breast-feeding. If supplies are inadequate, an unborn baby may leach calcium from its mother's body. Good dietary sources include leafy green vegetables like spinach and collard greens; broccoli; legumes such as soybeans, pinto beans, and black beans; and fish with soft, edible bones, such as herring and salmon. Calcium supplements may also be necessary, but consult with your obstetrician first.
- **Magnesium.** Necessary for the absorption of other minerals such as calcium. Magnesium also helps bones grow and teeth remain strong, keeps the body's metabolism in balance, and helps the muscles—including the heart—function properly. Women need 450 milligrams of magnesium daily

during pregnancy and while breast-feeding. Nutrition experts advise pregnant women to get magnesium from their diet rather than from supplements because of possible risks to their unborn babies. Good dietary sources include fish and seafood such as bluefish, cod, flounder, mackerel, and shrimp; leafy green vegetables; nuts; soybeans; and wheat germ.

- **Phosphorus.** Necessary for proper bone growth and maintenance, and instrumental to every chemical reaction that occurs in the body. Phosphorous also helps various tissues and systems utilize vitamins, fats, carbohydrates, and other nutrients. Women need 1,200 milligrams daily during pregnancy and breast-feeding. Good sources include lean red meat; calves' liver; poultry; seafood such as tuna, scallops, and canned sardines; dark green leafy vegetables; eggs and whole grain products.
- **Protein.** Necessary for proper fetal growth and development. Too little protein can result in stunted growth in children, as well as reduced immunological protection and a lack of energy. It is recommended that women consume 0.75 g of protein per kg of body weight a day during their first trimester (three months) of pregnancy and an additional 10 to 12 g a day for the second and third trimester. Good sources include poultry and lean meat, beans, and grains.
- **Vitamin D.** Necessary for the absorption of calcium and phosphorus, as well as the growth, hardening and repair of bones in both mother and child. Women 19 to 22 years of age need 1,000 IU daily during pregnancy and breast-feeding; women 23 and older need 800 IU during pregnancy and breast-

feeding. Good sources include oily fish with bones, such as herring and salmon; dark green leafy vegetables; liver; wheat germ; and whole grains. Sunlight is also important in the production of vitamin D, so make sure that you get adequate—but not excessive—sun exposure. Vitamin D supplements are also available, but make sure you get your doctor's approval before taking them because vitamin D can be toxic in high doses.

The following vitamins and minerals are not commonly found in dairy products but are also required by pregnant and breast-feeding women.

- **Folate** (also known as folic acid). 400 micrograms a day during pregnancy, 280 micrograms during the first six months of breast-feeding. Folate is essential in the prevention of certain birth defects and is considered vital before a woman becomes pregnant and during the first three months of pregnancy.
- **Iron.** 30 to 60 milligrams a day during pregnancy, 15 milligrams during the first six months of breast-feeding.
- **Niacin** (vitamin B_3). 17 milligrams a day during pregnancy, 20 milligrams during the first six months of pregnancy.
- **Vitamin A.** 800 micrograms a day during pregnancy, 1,300 micrograms during the first six months of pregnancy.
- **Vitamin C.** 70 milligrams a day during pregnancy, 95 milligrams during the first six months of breast-feeding.
- **Vitamin E.** 10 milligrams a day during pregnancy,

12 milligrams during the first six months of breast-feeding.
- **Zinc.** 15 milligrams a day during pregnancy, 19 milligrams during the first six months of pregnancy.

Q: I'm debating whether to breast-feed my new baby or give her a cow's milk-based commercial formula. Is cow's milk the nutritional equivalent of breast milk?

A: No. Cow's milk contains a lot of important nutrients, but nutrition experts say that it can't hold a candle to mother's milk and isn't interchangeable. If you have a choice, you should breast-feed your baby because breast milk is the most nutritious substance available.

The content of breast milk varies from woman to woman, and changes in composition to meet the needs of a baby as it grows. In general, however, it consists of water, fat, protein, sugars, vitamins, minerals, antibodies, and protective elements—everything a baby needs to grow and thrive. Breast-milk proteins are different from cow's-milk proteins. They form smaller curds and are generally easier for a baby to digest. In addition, the antibodies in breast milk destroy harmful bacteria and protect a newborn from infection during a period when its own immune system is still developing.

Another difference between breast milk and cow's milk is appearance. The first milk the breast produces is known as colostrum, and is low in fat and carbohydrates and high in protein. It tends to be thick and creamy in texture and contains protective antibodies. Following colostrum is transition milk, which tends to be thinner, and then mature milk, which is even thinner and sometimes bluish white in color.

Interestingly, note obstetricians, breast milk also

changes during each nursing session. The first milk that is produced is called the foremilk, which is the human equivalent of skim milk. Foremilk is followed by hindmilk, which is creamier and richer in proteins and fats.

Q: Both my husband and I are severely lactose intolerant, and we're afraid that our baby, which is due in two months, will be born with the condition. Is this possible?

A: There's a big difference between possible and likely. It's possible that your baby could be born lactose intolerant, but it's likely that it won't be. Let me reiterate: Lactose intolerance is not a disease that can be transmitted from one person to another; it's a genetic condition that usually occurs over time. If your baby grows up to be lactose intolerant, it's because of your genes and nothing else.

Babies born lactose intolerant—a condition known medically as congenital lactose intolerance—are extraordinarily rare. It happens, but the number of cases that occur in the United States each year is amazingly small. In fact, they could probably be counted on one hand. The vast majority of healthy babies produce plenty of lactase and can easily tolerate mother's milk or cow's milk-based formulas. As they age, their tolerance for lactose may diminish, but newborns are programmed to thrive on mother's milk (or a commercial substitute) because it's such a superior food.

As noted in Chapter Two, most babies in the past born with congenital lactose intolerance died within days because they couldn't tolerate the only food source available to them. However, doctors can now test for this condition at birth and provide a nutritious nondairy formula (often based on soy milk) for those rare babies that test positive.

A more common problem among newborns and young children is an allergy or intolerance to cow's milk protein. This problem most commonly affects newborns who are placed on a commercial formula based on cow's milk, or older children who receive cow's milk as part of their regular diet. Luckily, there are several nutritious infant formulas made from soy protein or hydrolyzed protein that can be used in place of cow's milk-based formulas. Soy-based products include Isomil, Nursoy, ProSobee, and Soylac. Hydrolyzed protein formulas include Nutramigen, Alimentum, and Pregestimil. Your pediatrician can provide more information on these special formulas if necessary. An allergy to cow's-milk protein can usually be controlled in older children by eliminating all dairy from their diets and making sure they receive proper nutrition through other dietary sources as well as supplements, if required.

Q: Can a baby be born allergic to its mother's milk?
A: There are few absolutes in this world, so we don't want to give you an unequivocal no. However, the chances of a baby being born allergic specifically to its mother's milk is infinitesimal. If an allergy does occur, it's more likely to be an allergy to something passed in the mother's milk, not the milk itself. The most common allergen is cow's-milk protein, although substances from other allergy-causing foods can be passed along in mother's milk.

Q: I understand that congenital lactose intolerance is extremely rare. But can babies acquire secondary lactose intolerance? It would seem to me that ba-

**bies are at risk of most of the same condition
adults can get.**

A: Babies can develop secondary lactose intolerance
from a number of sources. Some of the more serious
causes can result in permanent lactose intolerance, but
the majority of cases are temporary.

The most common causes of secondary lactose intolerance in infants are gastrointestinal infection or damage
to the intestines from disease or injury. Gastrointestinal
infection resulting in chronic diarrhea is by far the most
prevalent trigger, but the resulting lactose intolerance is
rarely permanent.

Babies older than six months are very susceptible to
intestinal viruses, and diarrhea is a common side effect
(infants younger than six months who are breast-fed appear to have greater protection as a result of antibodies
found in breast milk). Viral infections can last for days
or weeks and are often very frightening for parents.
(Note: diarrhea in babies lasting more than two days
should always be evaluated by a doctor.) However, most
bouts of diarrhea stop as quickly as they started, and the
majority of babies are none the worse for wear as a
result. But occasionally parents try to get their babies
back on breast milk or formula, only to have the diarrhea
recur with a vengeance, often accompanied by gas and
bloating. The diagnosis: secondary lactose intolerance.
However, it is important to note the difference between
loose stools and diarrhea in babies and not to confuse
them. Loose, runny stools in babies—particularly in
those who are breast-fed—are normal. Diarrhea in babies that occurs as a result of a virus or a dietary problem
is usually liquid, sometimes contains mucus, and occurs
with greater frequency and volume than a baby's normal
bowel movements.

Lactose intolerance most often occurs in babies and toddlers because special viruses known as rotoviruses attack the lactase-producing cells on the intestinal villi (tiny projections in the intestine that absorb available nutrients), eventually resulting in a lactase deficiency. After the viral infection runs its course, the symptoms of lactose intolerance may occur as soon as the baby returns to its normal diet. The child is otherwise healthy, just unable to digest lactose as well as she used to. This can be very disconcerting to parents, but the condition is seldom permanent. As soon as new lactase-producing cells mature and go to work, the condition usually disappears.

In a small percentage of cases, however, lactase production does not return to its previous levels. This is especially common in youngsters whose background or race gives them a strong predisposition to reduced lactase production at an early age, such as Asian children or black children from Africa. Poor lactase production may also be the result of an intestinal infection so severe that the cells on the intestinal lining are permanently damaged. Lactase may still be produced, but not in sufficient quantities to digest the total amount of lactose consumed during the average meal.

Infants with long-term lactose intolerance usually do well on supplemented nondairy formulas with a soy base, but you should always talk with your pediatrician before placing your child on such a dietary regimen to make sure it's the best course of action. In addition, some companies, such as Mead Johnson & Company, offer a milk-based, lactose-free formula that provides the benefits of cow's milk without the feeding problems associated with lactose. You can get more information on these formulas, which are made differently than tradi-

tional lactose-reduced products, from your doctor or by
calling Mead Johnson & Company toll-free at 800-
222-9123. The company's web site address is
www.meadjohnson.com.

**Q: Are intestinal viruses the only cause of lactose in-
tolerance in very young children?**
A: No. Babies and toddlers, just like adults, can also
develop lactose intolerance from other causes, including
medications such as antibiotics; diseases such as celiac
disease, giardiasis, and cystic fibrosis; and intestinal surgery. In short, anything that deeply affects the intestines
and the lactase-producing cells. In some cases, lactose
intolerance is permanent. In others, it's only temporary.

**Q: I work in a pediatric AIDS ward and have noticed
that chronic diarrhea is a frequent side effect of
the disease. Can AIDS lead to lactose intolerance
in infants and toddlers?**
A: Yes. Gastrointestinal problems are common among
babies born with HIV, most of whom contract the virus
from their mothers. Chronic diarrhea is a frequent side
effect, and this can damage the intestinal lining to the
point where lactase production is greatly reduced. The
result: gas, bloating, and more diarrhea. If care isn't
taken, dehydration and malnutrition can result. Of
course, this is true of all infants with chronic diarrhea,
which is why bouts lasting more than two days should
be evaluated by a pediatrician.

**Q: My sister's seven-month-old daughter is very col-
icky. She's fussy, cries constantly, and is difficult
to calm. Could lactose intolerance be the cause?**
A: Probably not. Colic, or gassiness, is frequently

caused by food, but rarely by lactose intolerance. The most common causes are garlic, onions, turnips, cabbage, prunes, beans, and excessive amounts of fruit. The condition can also result from caffeine or alcohol in mother's milk, which is one reason why new mothers are encouraged to avoid both until they are no longer breast-feeding. Some studies suggest that colic can be caused by maternal intake of cow's milk, which may induce colic in babies who have cow's milk protein intolerance. (See Chapter Three for more information on this condition.) Also, other studies show that maternal intake of certain foods, particularly cruciferous vegetables, may also be a cause of colic in some babies. Lactose intolerance is low on the list because researchers have tried giving colicky babies lactase drops and lactose-reduced milk with little reduction in fussiness or crying.

Your sister may be able to determine the cause of her daughter's colic by keeping a food journal and noting which foods appear to cause the child intestinal distress. She can then confirm the cause of the colic by eliminating that food for a while and monitoring her baby's behavior.

Q: How common is lactose intolerance among older children?

A: More common than most people assume. Lactose intolerance is generally regarded as an adult condition because it tends to be more obvious as people get older. But lactose intolerance can also afflict children and adolescents, especially those with a predisposition based on race or heritage. In cases such as these, lactose intolerance may begin to manifest in children as young as six or seven years.

As with pregnant and breast-feeding women, children with lactose intolerance are at risk of poor nutrition if appropriate substitutes aren't found for dairy products. Calcium is a special concern because growing children need plenty of the essential mineral for strong bones and teeth. As a result, parents must make sure that their children with lactose intolerance receive plenty of calcium-containing foods, such as leafy green vegetables and soybeans. Vitamin and mineral supplements may also be necessary.

Q: Is lactose intolerance substantially different in children than adults?
A: No. The condition is pretty much the same regardless of age. The most common symptoms—gas, bloating, and diarrhea—and their range of severity are the same in children as adults, though children are more likely than adults to also vomit as a result of dairy consumption. In addition, diagnostic tests for lactose intolerance are as effective on children as adults, as is dietary management and other available treatments for the condition.

Q: My 15-year-old son has moderate lactose intolerance diagnosed with a breath hydrogen test. Can he take lactase pills, or should he try to manage his condition by carefully monitoring his diet?
A: There's no reason your son can't take lactase pills with his meals. Lactase isn't a drug; it's a harmless enzyme naturally produced in the body and thus safe for people of all ages. You can't take too much of it, and it has no known side effects. According to pediatricians, lactase supplements, lactase drops for milk, and reduced-lactose dairy products can be given to infants the moment they go off formula and onto solid food.

Q: My 13-year-old daughter has lactose intolerance, and it's making her life miserable. She's doing poorly in school and refuses to make friends. How can we help her cope with her condition?

A: Lactose intolerance is usually much easier for adults to handle than children because adults are better able to understand the condition, its causes, and management. You can explain the condition to children until you're blue in the face, but in the end all they understand is that lactose intolerance may make them "different" from most of their friends and schoolmates—a situation that can be very difficult to cope with during a time when conformity is everything.

Helping your daughter deal with lactose intolerance will require compassion and understanding. The symptoms of the condition can be painful and embarrassing, especially if they happen at school or in front of friends, and many children cope by withdrawing into themselves.

Assuming that your daughter has been accurately diagnosed, it's up to you and your daughter's pediatrician to explain in terms she can understand what causes the condition and how it can be managed. Education is important—the more your daughter knows about lactose intolerance, the better able she'll be to deal with it. If you know someone who is lactose intolerant, ask them to sit down with your daughter and discuss the condition and how they handle it. Hearing about a problem from someone who's been there can be very enlightening.

Family members, close friends, and your daughter's teachers should be made aware of her condition and the fact that her diet is somewhat restricted. Outside of that group, however, there's really no reason for anyone to know that your daughter is lactose intolerant. When dining out with friends, she can select obvious nondairy foods and/or take lactase pills to prevent the onset of symptoms. Educate your daughter about which foods contain lactose—particularly foods that may contain hidden lactose—so that she will know which foods may cause symptoms of lactose intolerance. It would probably also be a good idea for your daughter to conduct a self-test to determine exactly how much lactose she can consume before symptoms occur, so she'll know her personal limits.

Most importantly, don't make your daughter's lactose intolerance a big issue. Refrain from discussing your daughter's condition with strangers or casual acquaintances, and make sure that siblings and friends don't tease her about it. With time, she'll come to realize that being lactose intolerant makes her part of the majority—not the minority—and that it's really nothing to worry or get upset about. (See Chapter Seven for more tips on coping with lactose intolerance.)

Q: I'm having trouble getting the staff at my son's school to recognize lactose intolerance and the need for a somewhat different menu for those children who have the condition. Any tips?

A: Many schools are attuned to the special needs of their students—including those with lactose intolerance. If the office and cafeteria staff at your son's school don't seem concerned, or refuse to honor your request for a selection of lactose-free foods, it may simply be that they don't know what lactose intolerance is, how pervasive it is, or how easy it can be to manage.

Schedule a meeting with the school principal and your son's instructors so you can educate them on lactose intolerance. Bring some literature with you to back up your concerns, then suggest ways that the school could help students with the condition. You can be fairly certain that a large percentage of your son's classmates are lactose intolerant to some degree, and your efforts will benefit them as well.

If the school administration still turns a deaf ear to your concerns, you may want to take the issue directly to your local school board. Organizing other parents of lactose-intolerant children will help bolster your cause. Again, make sure you back up your statements with authoritative evidence, such as this book.

Until the school listens to you and responds, your son can take lactase pills with his lunch (although you must make sure that you alert the school of your son's use of lactase pills, as many schools will not allow any medications to be brought in by students without clearance), select only those cafeteria foods he knows do not contain lactose, or bring his lunch from home. But don't despair. As the Baby Boomer generation ages, conditions such as lactose intolerance are receiving more and more publicity and public awareness. You should have little difficulty convincing the right people that lactose intolerance is widespread and needs to be addressed.

Q: After more than 60 years of problem-free dairy consumption, I was diagnosed with lactose intolerance. Is this a common condition among older Americans?

A: Lactose intolerance is a common condition among all Americans, but it has a relatively high prevalence among seniors—those 55 and older—because it tends to become more evident with age. Don't forget: Primary acquired lactose intolerance (the most common form of the condition) generally occurs gradually over many years. If you have a predisposition to the condition, as many people do, then it makes sense for symptoms to become more apparent during the later years as lactase production diminishes.

According to gerontologists (doctors who specialize in the health problems associated with aging), digestive problems in general are more common among older people. Disorders of the digestive tract cause more hospital admissions than any other group of diseases, research shows, and they most frequently afflict middle-aged and older adults.

Very often, the physical effects of aging are to blame. If a person has difficulty chewing, for example, she may avoid high-fiber foods such as corn and apples in favor of soft, processed meals such as macaroni and cheese or pudding. This can lead to constipation and other digestive problems, which are often made worse by a lack of exercise and low fluid intake. The stomach's ability to produce enough acid for proper digestion also decreases with age, resulting in still more digestive difficulties.

Luckily, almost all of these problems can be managed fairly easily. People who have difficulty chewing because of ill-fitting dentures or other problems can still get plenty of fiber in their diet by eating softer alternatives such as oatmeal, stewed or canned fruits, beans, steamed vegetables, brown rice, and salad. Digestive problem can also be avoided by drinking plenty of water every day, and exercising regularly—even if it's just a walk around the block.

If chronic heartburn is your problem, avoid rich or spicy foods. This includes the obvious, such as Mexican food or chili, but also common dishes such as tomato products, chocolate, and fried foods. It also helps to eat small, frequent meals; drink plenty of water with your meals; and sit up for a few hours after eating. Lying down immediately after a meal can promote a painful backwash of stomach acid into the esophagus.

Most importantly, don't hesitate to see a doctor if you notice any distinct changes in your digestive or bowel habits. Many digestive problems can be serious, but are usually easy to treat if detected early.

Q: What are the most common concerns regarding lactose intolerance in the elderly?

A: As with pregnant women, the biggest concern regarding lactose intolerance in the elderly is adequate nutrition. The easiest response to lactose intolerance is to avoid the foods that cause symptoms. However, milk and other dairy products are a big source of essential nutrients, including calcium, and poor nutrition may result if dairy products are not replaced with nutritionally equivalent substitutes.

Pregnant women need calcium, vitamin D, magnesium, and other nutrients to ensure good health for themselves and healthy growth and development for their babies. Older people need these nutrients, too, to maintain bone strength and ward off debilitating osteoporosis. You'll recall from Chapter Six that osteoporosis is extremely common among older people—especially women—and can result in brittle bones and potentially crippling fractures. However, it's never too late to add more calcium and other nutrients to your diet. The best calcium comes from the foods we eat, but older people may also require supplements. Make sure you discuss supplementation with your doctor before beginning such a regimen.

Another concern regarding lactose intolerance and the elderly is the potential for dehydration from chronic diarrhea. Older people with the condition may not realize that their symptoms result from the consumption of lactose and continue to eat dairy products under the mistaken belief that their digestive problems are just a normal part of aging. However, diarrhea can quickly deplete the body of fluids and adversely affect almost every organ and system, so drink as much liquid as you can. (Contrary to popular belief, avoiding liquids will not reduce the severity or longevity of a diarrhea attack. It will only hurt your body more.) Water is good, but beverages designed for athletes, such as Gatorade, can also be beneficial. Diarrhea lasting more than a couple of days should be evaluated by a doctor.

The management of lactose intolerance among the elderly is fairly easy. As with other populations, those with the condition can usually consume small amounts of dairy and are encouraged to eat as much as their systems will allow in an effort to maintain good nutrition. In addition, lactase pills can be taken with meals, and lactose-reduced dairy products offer a safe alternative to regular dairy. Seniors should also read food labels carefully to make sure they're not consuming hidden lactose, which is a very common problem with processed foods. (See Chapter Seven for a more definitive discussion of the dairy-indicative words to watch out for, as well as other management tips.)

Q: I'm 68 and take a large number of medications each day as a result of various health problems. I also have lactose intolerance. A good friend of mine told me that my pills could actually lead to the onset of symptoms. Should I be concerned?

A: The answer is yes and no. As noted in Chapter Seven, many pharmaceutical companies add lactose to their pills and capsules because it makes a great filler or base. Lactose doesn't clump or cake, it dissolves almost immediately, and is considered safe and nontoxic. In theory, the inclusion of lactose in prescription and over-the-counter medications could trigger symptoms in people with lactose intolerance. However, the amount used is generally so small as to be inconsequential for the majority of people with the condition.

Those most at risk are people such as you—older individuals who consume a large number of pills each day for the management of various medical conditions. According to government health officials, more than three-fourths of Americans 65 and older regularly take at least one prescription medication, and many take several. It's possible that the cumulative amount of lactose from your medications could result in symptoms, though this is extremely rare and occurs only in cases of extreme lactose intolerance. Unless your condition is so severe that you become ill from the smallest amounts of lactose, you should have little to worry about. However, if the issue still bothers you, talk with your doctor about lactose-free alternatives.

Q: My wife has muscular multiple sclerosis, which she manages fairly well. She is also lactose intolerant. We were both wondering: Can lactose intolerance have an impact on multiple sclerosis or any other chronic illnesses?

A: Generally, no. Lactose intolerance affects only the digestive system—specifically the intestines—and rarely influences any other organ or body system. As a result, most people with common chronic illnesses who are also lactose intolerant find that the condition seldom affects their specific disease.

Sometimes, however, a chronic disorder may result in

lactose intolerance as a secondary condition. This occurs most often in people who have diseases of the digestive system, such as Crohn's disease, though it may also occur as a result of diseases not generally associated with the digestive system, such as cystic fibrosis, AIDS, and diabetes. The management of secondary lactose intolerance is pretty much the same as for primary acquired lactose intolerance. (See Chapter Four.)

One final note: Lactose intolerance can have a detrimental effect on nutrition, especially if a person avoids all dairy products and doesn't replace them with alternative sources of essential vitamins and minerals. Poor nutrition can greatly affect the management and treatment of many chronic diseases, so individuals with long-term conditions who are also lactose intolerant should discuss this issue with their doctors to make sure they are eating as well as possible. If necessary, your doctor may suggest nutritional supplements to give your body an extra boost.

Glossary

alactasia—a medical term for a lactase deficiency.

alimentary canal—the digestive tract extending from the mouth to the anus.

autonomic nervous system—the sympathetic and parasympathetic divisions of the nervous system that control the motor functions of the heart, lungs, intestines, glands and other internal organs.

borborygmi—rumbling sounds made by gas and fluid in the intestines. A common symptom of lactose intolerance.

bowel resection—the surgical removal of part or all of the small or large intestine.

casein—a protein that is one of the chief constituents of milk and the basis of cheese.

celiac sprue—a genetic condition characterized by an inability to digest a grain protein known as gluten. Symptoms of gas, bloating and diarrhea often mimic those of lactose intolerance. Also called celiac disease.

chyme—the thick, semifluid mass resulting from gastric digestion of food.

congenital lactose intolerance—an extremely rare condition in which a baby is born without the ability to naturally produce lactase.

cow's milk protein allergy—a reaction by the immune system to whey or casein proteins in cow's milk.

differential diagnosis—a technique of diagnosing illness by methodically eliminating potential ailments until only the correct one remains.

endoscopy—a procedure for looking into hollow organs of the body via a miniature television camera. Useful in diagnosing diseases of the colon and stomach.

enzymes—proteins that act as catalysts in the numerous chemical reactions that occur in living things. Lactase is an enzyme.

galactosemia—a potentially dangerous congenital disease caused by the lack of an enzyme necessary for the metabolization of galactose, one of the two simple sugars that combine to create lactose.

gastroenterology—the study of the digestive system and its diseases.

gerontologist—a doctor who deals with the health problems associated with aging.

glycolysis—the breakdown of sugars or other carbohydrates by enzymes into simpler compounds.

inflammatory bowel disease—an umbrella term for a number of gastrointestinal diseases commonly characterized by gas, bloating, diarrhea and other symptoms. Crohn's disease and ulcerative colitis are examples of inflammatory bowel disease.

kosher—a designation given to foods deemed fit to eat

according to Jewish dietary laws and rituals. Kosher foods often contain no dairy and are helpful in the management of lactose intolerance. (See also *pareve*.)

lactase—an enzyme produced in the intestines necessary for the breakdown and digestion of lactose.

lactase deficiency—a shortage of lactase in the intestines.

lactic acid—a substance produced by the fermentation of lactose when milk sours. A common side product in the manufacture of yogurt.

lactose—the sugar found in the milk of nearly all mammals. Lactose is made by combining two simple sugars, glucose and galactose.

lactose intolerance—a common condition characterized by an inability to digest lactose because of diminishing amounts of lactase in the intestines. Symptoms commonly include gas, bloating, and diarrhea. Most cases are age-related (primary acquired lactose intolerance or adult-onset lactose intolerance).

lactose maldigestion (also known as lactose malabsorption)—the inability to digest lactose, caused by either a natural reduction in lactase production, damage to the intestines, or conditions that prevent lactose from being exposed to lactase for sufficient periods. May or may not be accompanied by common symptoms of lactose intolerance.

osteoporosis—a common disease characterized by weak, brittle, easily broken bones. Osteoporosis results when calcium levels in the diet are insufficient to maintain bone density. Most often seen in postmenopausal women.

pareve—foods designated as "neutral" under Jewish dietary law because they contain no meat or dairy products. Can be helpful in the management of lactose intolerance.

pasteurization—a method of destroying disease-producing bacteria in liquids such as milk or beer by heating the liquid to a prescribed temperature for a specific period of time.

peristalsis—muscle contractions that move food through the digestive system.

secondary lactose intolerance—a form of lactose intolerance caused by the use of certain medications or disease or injury to the intestines. The condition can be temporary or permanent.

villi—The numerous hairlike or fingerlike projections that cover certain mucous membranes in the body, including the small intestine.

whey—the liquid that remains during the manufacture of cheese. Whey is very high in lactose and should be avoided by individuals with lactose intolerance.

Resource Organizations

American Academy of Allergy, Asthma and Immunology, 611 East Wells Street, Milwaukee, WI 53202. Phone: 414-272-6071. Physicians' Referral and Information Line: 800-822-2762.

American Cancer Society, 1599 Clifton Road, NE, Atlanta, GA 30329. Phone: 800-227-2345.

American Dairy Products Institute, 300 West Washington Street, Suite 400, Chicago, IL 60606. Phone: 312-782-4888.

American Dietetic Association, 216 West Jackson Boulevard, Suite 800, Chicago, IL 60606. Phone: 312-899-0040. Nutrition Hot Line and Referrals: 800-366-1655.

Digestive Disease National Coalition, 507 Capitol Court NE, Suite 200, Washington, DC 20002. Phone: 202-544-7497.

Food Allergy Network, 10400 Eaton Place, Suite 107, Fairfax, VA 22030. Phone: 800-929-4040.

National Cancer Institute, Cancer Information Service (CIS), Building 31, Room 10A24, Bethesda, MD 20892. Phone: 800-422-6237.

National Digestive Diseases Education and Information Clearinghouse, 2 Information Way, Bethesda, MD 20892. Phone: 301-654-3810.

National Foundation for Ileitis and Colitis/Crohn's and Colitis Foundation of America, 386 Park Avenue South, 17th Floor, New York, NY 10016. Phone: 800-343-3637.

National Osteoporosis Foundation, 1150 17th Street NW, Suite 500, Washington, DC 20037. Phone: 202-223-2226.

National Yogurt Association, 2000 Corporate Ridge, Suite 1000, McLean, VA 22102. Phone: 703-821-0770.

Bibliography

Adverse Reactions to Foods, American Academy of Allergy and Immunology. Milwaukee, WI: American Academy of Allergy and Immunology, 1994.

Blue Ribbon Babies: Eating Well During Pregnancy, American Dietetic Association. Chicago, IL: American Dietetic Association, 1989.

The Breastfeeding Answer Book, N. Mohrbacher, J. Stock. Franklin Park, IL: La Leche League International, 1991.

The Columbia University School of Public Health Complete Guide to Health and Well-Being After 50, R.J. Weiss, Subak-Sharpe, J. Genell, Editors. New York, NY: Times Books, 1988.

The Complete Book of Cancer Prevention, C. Keough, Editor. Emmaus, PA: Rodale Press, 1988.

The Complete Book of Children's Allergies: A Guide for Parents, B.R. Feldman, D. Carroll. New York, NY: Times Books, 1986.

The Complete Book of Pregnancy and Childbirth, S. Kitzinger. New York, NY: Knopf, 1989.

The Complete Guide to Food Allergy and Intolerance: Prevention, Identification, and Treatment of Common Illnesses and Allergies Caused by Food, J. Brostoff, L. Gamlin. New York, NY: Crown, 1989.

The Doctor's Complete Guide to Vitamins and Minerals, M. Eades. New York, NY: Dell, 1994.

Don't Drink Your Milk, 9th edition, F.A. Oski. Brushton, NY: TEACH Services, 1983.

Eating for Two: The Complete Guide to Nutrition During Pregnancy, M. Hess, A. Hunt. New York, NY: Macmillan, 1992.

Food Allergies, M.L. Dobler. Chicago, IL: National Center for Nutrition and Dietetics of the American Dietetic Association, 1993.

Food—Your Miracle Medicine, J. Carper. New York, NY: HarperCollins, 1993.

Hidden Food Allergies, S. Astor. Garden City Park, NY: Avery Publishing Group, 1988.

How Strong Are Your Bones? Washington, DC: National Osteoporosis Foundation, 1994.

Infant Nutrition and Feeding, Food and Nutrition Service. Washington, DC: U.S. Department of Agriculture, 1993.

Lactose Intolerance, M.L. Dobler. Chicago, IL: National Center for Nutrition and Dietetics of the American Dietetic Association, 1992.

Medical Management of Non-insulin-dependent (Type II) Diabetes, 3rd ed., American Diabetes Association. Alexandria, VA: 1994.

Menopause, Washington, DC: National Women's Health Resource Center, 1993.

The Menopause Handbook, S.F. Trien. New York, NY: Ballantine Books, 1986.

Menopause Naturally: Preparing for the Second Half of Life, S. Greenwood. Volcano, CA: Volcano Press, 1989.

The Menopause Years. Washington, DC: American College of Obstetricians and Gynecologists, 1992.

Milk is Not for Every Body: Living with Lactose Intolerance, S. Carper. New York, NY: Plume Books, 1996.

The Milk Sugar Dilemma: Living with Lactose Intolerance, R.A. Martens, S. Martens. East Lansing, MI: Medi-Ed Press, 1987.

Nutrition and Diet Therapy, 6th edition, C. Townsend. Albany, NY: Delmar Publishers, Inc., 1994.

The Nutrition Desk Reference, R. Garrison, E. Somer. New Canaan, CT: Keats Publishing, 1990.

Nutrition During Pregnancy and Lactation: An Implementation Guide, Committee on Nutritional Status During Pregnancy and Lactation, Food and Nutrition Board, Institute of Medicine, National Academy of Sciences. Washington, DC: National Academy Press, 1992.

Nutrition for Your Pregnancy: The University of Minnesota Guide, J. Brown. Minneapolis, MN: University of Minnesota Press, 1983.

The PDR Family Guide to Nutrition and Health, D. Sifton, Editor. Montvale, NJ: Medical Economics Company, 1995.

Pediatric Nutrition Handbook, L. Barnes, Editor. Elk Grove Village, IL: American Academy of Pediatrics, 1993.

Planning for Pregnancy, Birth, and Beyond, American

College of Obstetricians and Gynecologists. New York, NY: Dutton, 1992.

Stand Up to Osteoporosis, Washington, DC: National Osteoporosis Foundation, 1992.

The Tufts University Guide to Total Nutrition, S. Gershoff, C. Whitney. New York, NY: Harper & Row, 1990.

Your Food-Allergic Child: A Parent's Guide, J. Meizel. Bedford, MA: Mills & Sanderson, 1988.

Informative Web Sites

Lehigh Valley Hospital and Health Network: *www.lvhhn.org*

Living With Ulcerative Colitis: Insights and Answers for Better Living: *www.living-better.com*

National Digestive Diseases Education and Information Clearinghouse: *www.niddk.nih.gov*

National Osteoporosis Foundation: *www.nof.org*

Steve Carper's Homepage (Carper has written extensively about lactose intolerance): *www.ourworld. compuserve.com/homepages/stevecarper*

Union of Orthodox Jewish Congregations of America (includes much information on kosher foods, including those that are free of dairy products): *www.ou.org*

Index

A native of Mexico City, Mexico, JAIME ARANDA-MICHEL, M.D., completed his medical degree at the School of Medicine, Universidad Nacional, Autonoma de Mexico, in Mexico City. He has taken additional training in Australia, at the Mayo Foundation in Minnesota, and at the University of Alabama at Birmingham, and is board certified in gastroenterology, internal medicine, hepatology, and nutrition. Dr. Aranda-Michel is currently a senior fellow in gastroenterolgy in the Division of Digestive Diseases at the University of Cincinnati, Ohio. He resides in Cincinnati.

DONALD S. VAUGHAN is a North Carolina-based freelance writer who specializes in health and medical issues. His work has appeared in dozens of publications, including *Omni*, *Modern Maturity*, and *Your Health* magazines.

THE NEW YORK TIMES FOUR-MILLION-COPY BESTSELLER

DR. ATKINS' NEW DIET REVOLUTION

THE AMAZING NO-HUNGER WEIGHT-LOSS PLAN THAT HAS HELPED MILLIONS LOSE WEIGHT AND KEEP IT OFF

by Robert C. Atkins, M.D.

72729-3/$6.99 US/$8.99 Can

Alternative Healing Approaches

KAVA
NATURE'S STRESS RELIEF
by Kathryn M. Connor, M.D. and Donald S. Vaughan
80641-X/$5.99 US/$7.99 Can

ST. JOHN'S WORT
NATURE'S MOOD BOOSTER
*Everything You Need to Know about This
Natural Antidepressant*
by Michael E. Thase, M.D. and Elizabeth E. Loredo
80288-0/$5.99 US/$7.99 Can

GINKGO
NATURE'S BRAIN BOOSTER
by Alan H. Pressman, D.C., Ph.D., C.C.N.
with Helen Tracy
80640-1/$5.99 US/$7.99 Can

A HANDBOOK OF NATURAL FOLK REMEDIES
by Elena Oumano, Ph.D.
78448-3/$5.99 US/$7.99 Can